THE EXTREME ENDOMORPH DIET AND EXERCISE PLAN FOR BEGINNERS

Metabolism Mastery: The Comprehensive Guide to Energizing Nutrition and Easy Fitness for Every Body Type - Fast, Delicious, and Balanced Recipes with Optimized Exercises for Men, Women and Seniors

Vincent John Walker

1

DISCLAIMER

This publication is designed to provide competent and reliable information regarding the subject covered. However, the views expressed in this publication are those of the author alone, and should not be taken as expert instruction or professional advice. The reader is responsible for his or her actions. The author hereby disclaims any responsibility or liability whatsoever that is incurred from the use or application of the contents of this publication by the purchaser of the reader. The purchaser or reader is hereby responsible for his or her actions.

Copyright © 2024

TABLE OF CONTENTS

INTRODUCTION

This isn't just another fitness book; it's a groundbreaking journey tailored for the endomorph body type, aimed at sculpting a healthier, fitter, and more vibrant you.

In a fitness world cluttered with one-size-fits-all advice, it's time to celebrate our unique differences. The key to unlocking lasting health and fitness success isn't found in following the crowd but in understanding and embracing our individuality—our unique body shapes, sizes, and metabolic rhythms.

For those with an endomorph physique—naturally fuller, more voluptuous, and inclined to store fat—the path to wellness can seem fraught with challenges. But what if these perceived hurdles are stepping stones to greater strength, confidence, and well-being? "ENDOMORPH REVOLUTION" is not just a guide; it's a movement towards embracing and optimizing your natural body type to achieve your wellness goals.

Dive into a treasure trove of cutting-edge insights, where we decode the science of the endomorph body. This book is a beacon, illuminating the path to understanding your genetic blueprint and metabolic idiosyncrasies. It's about transforming knowledge into power—the power to love your body set actionable goals, and tailor a lifestyle that's in harmony with your nature.

Our mission is bold yet simple: to equip you with a toolkit brimming with effective strategies, empowering you to unleash your endomorph potential. Whether your vision is shedding unwanted weight, sculpting muscle, elevating your energy levels, or simply embracing a healthier way of living, this guide is your ally.

Prepare to be introduced to a world where nutrition isn't about restriction but about strategic choices that thrill your palate while fueling your body. Where exercise goes beyond repetitive routines to become a catalyst for change, designed with your unique body type in mind.

"THE EXTREME ENDOMORPH DIET AND EXERCISE PLAN FOR BEGINNERS" transcends the ordinary, offering a holistic vista that includes rest, recovery, and mastering the art of stress management. It's a guide that understands life's ups and downs, teaching you to navigate challenges, celebrate progress, and stay motivated through every season of your journey.

Featuring inspiring stories from real people who've walked this path and transformed their lives, this book is a testament to what's possible when you receive the right guidance, infused with determination and support.

So, as we embark on this transformative adventure together, remember: that being an endomorph is your superpower. With "ENDOMORPH REVOLUTION" as your guide, you're not just chasing a goal; you're unlocking a lifestyle where achieving your dream health and vitality is not only possible but inevitable.

Are you ready to revolutionize your life? "ENDOMORPH REVOLUTION: THE BEGINNER'S DIET & WORKOUT BLUEPRINT" is your first step towards a triumphant journey to the best version of yourself. Let the revolution begin.

BASIC ENDOMORPH

What Does an Endomorph Mean?

One of the three fundamental somatotypes, or body types, used to categorize and characterize variations in human morphology is the endomorph. The idea of somatotypes was developed in the 1940s by American psychologist William H. Sheldon as a way to group individuals according to their physical characteristics and body composition.

Understanding Your Body Type: Endomorph

In the fascinating field of human biology, there is a remarkable diversity of body kinds, each with unique traits, capacities, and issues. One such body type is the endomorph, which differs from its relatives who are ectomorphic and mesomorphic in several essential ways. Since it provides a foundation for individualized solutions, understanding the endomorph body type is the first step in achieving optimum health and fitness.

Features of Endomorphs:

Compared to other body types, endomorphs are genetically predisposed to store body fat more rapidly. When faced with a calorie excess, endomorphs are more prone to gain fat in areas like the belly, hips, and thighs.

Endomorphs have a rounder face, a wider body, and a softer, curvier appearance. They could have a more pronounced apple or pear-shaped profile and be smaller in height.

Slower Metabolism: Metabolism is the rate at which the body uses energy from calories. Compared to ectomorphs, endomorphs have a slower metabolic rate (those with a slimmer physique). This suggests that to maintain or lose weight, people may need to exercise more consistently and be more aware of their calorie intake.

Endomorphs may put on a lot of muscle mass even if they are more likely to accumulate body fat. With the right exercise program, they might gain strength and definition in their physique.

Oftentimes, endomorphs find it more difficult to gain weight than those with other body types. This might be a blessing and a curse since it implies they could increase muscle mass quickly if they use the right approach, but they also have to watch what they eat and how much they exercise to prevent gaining unwanted body fat.

Acceptance of Endomorph Body Type:

It is important to emphasize that being an endomorph is a unique quality with its advantages rather than a drawback. Once you are aware of your body type, you may modify your fitness and health regimens to accommodate your genetic predispositions. Here are a few important things to keep in mind:

Endomorphs tend to accumulate fat, so they should be very mindful of what they eat. Restricting calories while maintaining a nutrient-dense, well-balanced diet may help with weight control.

Strength Training Is Crucial: Endomorphs are excellent at building muscle and gaining strength. Resistance training can improve your body composition and speed up your metabolism when added to your exercise regimen.

Cardiovascular exercise: For overall health and calorie expenditure, cardiovascular activity is just as important as strength training. Finding a balance between the two types of exercise is essential.

Endomorphs may need more time to reach their fitness and health goals, but perseverance and patience are crucial. Changes that are gradual yet significant might result in big changes.

The Benefits of Customized Methods

When it comes to fitness and wellness, there is no one-size-fits-all solution. Personalized or customized tactics, often referred to as bespoke strategies, are essential for ensuring long-term success, inspiring staff, and producing the greatest results. These methods evaluate the specific characteristics, needs, goals, and constraints of each person rather than relying on universally applicable answers. Personalized approaches are crucial for the following reasons:

- **Increasing Effectiveness:** Everybody is different in terms of their genetics, metabolism, body type, degree of fitness, and health. What functions effectively for one person may not be as effective for another. A customized approach considers each of these unique factors to create a plan that maximizes effectiveness.

- **Getting Long-Term Results:** Most of the time, diet and exercise regimens that are generic work well in the short term but fall short in the long run. A customized strategy takes into account a person's preferences, way of life, and constraints, which raises the possibility that they will stick to the plan over time.

- **Preventing Accidents and Health Risks:** Injuries and health risks may arise from forcing individuals to engage in activities or follow diets that are unsuitable for their physical capabilities. Tailored methods provide safety by accounting for an individual's physical limitations, health status, and degree of fitness.

- **When a plan is customized**, people are more likely to remain motivated because they see results that are pertinent to their objectives. This improves compliance and raises the likelihood of reaching and maintaining desired outcomes.

- **Changing Needs:** Goals for fitness, health issues, and life situations may all change over time. A customized approach may be easily modified to accommodate these changes while maintaining its efficacy and applicability.

- **Considering Psychological Aspects:** Customized methods may also include psychological elements, such as an individual's inclinations, way of thinking, and emotional connection to exercise and eating. Although these components are sometimes overlooked in general tactics, they are essential to long-term success.

- **Resource and Time Optimization:** Not everyone has the same resources or time available to them. Because it takes into account a person's time constraints, financial situation, and access to resources, a customized approach is more feasible and practical.

- **Enhancing General Well-Being:** Fitness and health should be about more than simply appearance or output. A more holistic and pleasurable trip may be achieved by using a tailored strategy that considers all aspects of an individual's well-being, including mental health, stress levels, and quality of life.

- **Personal Empowerment:** By taking part in the creation of a personalized plan, people feel more in control of their health and fitness. A feeling of ownership and accountability for one's well-being is fostered by this empowerment.

- Good healthcare and fitness practices are built on the ethical principle of recognizing and acknowledging the uniqueness of persons and their unique needs.

PLANNING YOUR GOALS

The Process of Determining Your Health and Fitness Goals

To take the first step toward a healthier and more active lifestyle, it is essential to lay down your objectives for health and fitness. Having well-defined objectives provides you with a sense of direction, motivation, and a framework for arranging your fitness and health program. When it comes to determining your health and fitness objectives, here is a comprehensive guide:

Personal Contemplation:

- assessing your current level of health and fitness is the first step in determining your preexisting health status. It is important to take into consideration your weight, body composition, blood pressure, cholesterol levels, and any other conditions that you may be experiencing. By doing this baseline exam, you will be able to determine your current position more accurately.

- Among the physical traits that should be taken into consideration are things like strength, flexibility, endurance, and balance. Compile a list of any limitations or areas in which you would want to see improvements for yourself.

- Take some time to think about the routines you follow daily, such as your eating habits, your workout routine, your sleeping patterns, and how you deal with stress. Examine the areas in which you have room for development.

Determine Particular Objectives:

- Ensure that your goals are communicated clearly and precisely. Rather than stating a generic target such as "lose weight," you should specify the amount of weight you want to lose and the time frame in which you want to lose it.

- The goals that you set for yourself should be measurable so that you can track your progress. Measures such as weight reduction, inches gained, or the number of times you exercise should be used.

- It is important to ensure that your goals are not just attainable but also realistic. To position yourself for success, you should establish objectives that are within your grasp.

- If you want your goals to be relevant, they should be connected to your life and your principles. They should be on the priorities that you have.

- Time-bound: Give each of your objectives a start date and an end date. This not only helps you feel more accountable, but it also gives you a feeling of urgency. One example would be to establish a goal of obtaining a certain level of fitness within three months.

Investigate several Different Aspects of Health and Fitness:

- To improve your physical fitness, you need to set certain objectives for yourself, such as boosting your cardiovascular endurance, strength, flexibility, or balance.

- Identify specific dietary objectives, such as reducing the amount of sugar you consume, increasing the number of meals you prepare at home, or eating a certain number of servings of fruits and vegetables daily.

- The management of weight: If you are worried about your weight, you should set weight-related goals for yourself, such as reducing a certain number of pounds or maintaining a healthy weight range.

- Take care of your mental and emotional health; you should not ignore the importance of these aspects of your life. Take into consideration activities that can help you reduce stress, enhance your sleep, or practice mindfulness.

Establish Your Goals in Priority Order:

- Sort your objectives following the relevance of each one. You will be able to concentrate on the most critical objectives while avoiding overload as a result of this.

Formulate a plan of action:

- Put your goals into more achievable chunks by breaking them down into smaller activities. For instance, if you want to run a marathon, you may begin by participating in a couch-to-5k program, gradually increase the number of kilometers you run, and do this by taking part in smaller events as milestones along the way.
- Take into account the amount of time, money, and help that will be necessary to achieve each aim.

Observe and Make Adjustments:

- Your progress may be monitored regularly by using a spreadsheet, a fitness app, or a journal. Maintain a record of both your successes and your setbacks.
- Always be open to making adjustments. You should adjust a goal following the circumstances if you find that it is either too difficult or not challenging enough.

Remain Responsible and Accountable:

- One of your friends, a member of your family, or a coach who can assist you in staying on track should be informed of your goals.
- Consider becoming a member of an exercise club, a class, or an online community to get additional support and motivation.

Celebrate Significant Milestones:

- You should celebrate your achievements at various points along the way. Be sure to acknowledge and praise yourself when you reach a significant milestone, but steer clear of using food as a reward.

Reevaluate and Establish New Objectives:

- It is important to frequently assess your progress and set new goals as you make progress toward achieving your initial objectives. You will remain motivated as a result of this, and it will ensure that you continue to develop and advance.

Providing Endomorphs with Realistic Objectives

It is essential for individuals of all body types, particularly endomorphs, to come up with attainable objectives. To achieve your health and fitness objectives as an endomorph, it is necessary to take into consideration the particular characteristics and constraints of your body. As an endomorph, the following are some guidelines that can assist you in developing goals that are attainable:

1. Acknowledge that your aims are reasonable:

- Be conscious of the fact that your development can be going more slowly than that of other body types. Because endomorphs tend to put on fat, it may take them a longer period to demonstrate visible effects from their efforts.

2. Pay attention to the composition of your body:

- Instead of concentrating just on weight reduction, you should search for changes in the makeup of your body. This involves raising the amount of lean muscle mass and decreasing the amount of body fat, both of which may lead to a more youthful look.

3. Establish both short-term and long-term goals according to the following:

- Create a series of smaller, more doable benchmarks that represent your final goal. This provides you with a feeling of accomplishment and helps you maintain your motivation along the way.

4. Establish SMART goals:

- Detailed: Clearly articulate the goals you want to achieve.

- The use of measurable metrics, such as the percentage of body fat or the amount of inches lost, is recommended.

- Setting objectives that are within your grasp, taking into consideration your body type and starting position, is an effective way to be able to achieve your goals.

- Make sure that your goals are in line with the things that are most important to you in terms of your health and fitness.

- Time-Bound: Establish a timeline that realistically allows you to accomplish each of your goals.

5. Focus on achieving victories on a manageable scale:

- It is important to recognize and honor achievements that go beyond the scale, such as higher levels of stamina, strength, flexibility, and total energy.

Ensure that nutrition is a top priority:

- Establish dietary goals that include eating in a balanced manner, managing portion sizes, and consuming healthier foods wherever possible.

A Method for Succeeding in Weight Loss:

- You should aim to drop between half a pound and one pound every week if you want to achieve your weight loss goals: moderate and steady. Rapid weight loss may lead to a loss of muscle mass as well as a slowdown in metabolism.

Include Strength Training in Your Routine:

- Establish objectives for your strength training and the development of your muscles. Endomorphs can effectively increase muscle, which may be beneficial for improving body composition and boosting metabolism.

Include cardiovascular exercise into your routine:

- To maintain a healthy heart and burn calories, cardiovascular activity is very necessary. Assist in the process of weight reduction by establishing goals for engaging in regular cardiovascular activity.

Monitor Your Advancement:

- To document your progress, you should take measurements, take images, and maintain a fitness diary. This makes it possible for you to recognize favorable advances even if they are not immediately available to you.

Be patient and consistent in your actions:

- Understand that progress is a process that requires time. Remain steadfast in your dedication to achieving your objectives, and have trust in the process.

Keeping track of what's happening and keeping oneself motivated

The ability to effectively assess your progress and maintain motivation are essential components in achieving your health and fitness objectives, regardless of the sort of body you find yourself in. As an endomorph, it is of the utmost importance to evaluate your progress consistently to motivate yourself and keep on course. Listed below are some strategies that can assist you in accurately measuring your progress and keeping your motivation levels high:

- Step one is to establish objectives that are both clear and detailed. Having goals that are both clear and well-defined will provide you with a distinct sense of purpose. Make sure that your goals are specific, quantifiable, realistic, relevant, and have a time threshold attached to them (SMART).

- Maintain a Fitness Journal: Keep a journal in which you document your workouts, the foods you eat, and your overall health and wellness. Throughout your path toward better health and fitness, this notebook might be of assistance to you in monitoring your progress and seeing patterns.

- Make sure to take measurements regularly: To monitor your physical changes, it is important to measure important factors such as your weight, body fat percentage, waist circumference, and muscle mass. Consistency in the settings under which measurements are taken (for instance, at the same time of day and wearing the same dress) ensures trustworthy findings.

- Keep note of milestones that are not measured by a scale: Celebrate victories that go beyond the numbers on the scale, such as improved endurance, strength, flexibility, and energy levels. Successes like this have the potential to serve as powerful motivators.

- Make Use of Technology: Utilize fitness apps, wearable devices, and online resources to keep track of your progress, calculate the number of calories you burn, and document the workouts you perform. There are a number of these tools that also provide graphically displayed representations of your progress, which may be incredibly motivating.

- Photographic Progress: Take pictures of yourself regularly, ensuring that the lighting and postures are constant so that you can visually follow the changes that occur in your body over time. The perception of physical improvements may be a potent motivator.

- Establish a Reward System: Establish a system in which you will reward yourself for accomplishing certain predetermined objectives. The prizes that you get should follow your fitness objectives (for example, you should refrain from using unhealthy foods as incentives). Some examples of these prizes are new workout equipment, a day at the spa, or an exciting adventure.

- Talk About Your Objectives Have a conversation with a friend, a member of your family, or a workout partner about your expectations for your health and fitness. You may be a great motivator by holding yourself accountable, and having someone with whom you can communicate both your triumphs and your challenges can help you remain interested in the activity.

- Participate in a Helpful Community: If you want to meet individuals who share your interests, you should join fitness forums, social media groups, or local fitness clubs. Through the formation of friendships and the provision of support, participation in a community may increase one's level of motivation.

NUTRITIONAL BENEFIT FOR ENDOMORPH

Endomorph-Specific Requirements in Nutrition

Endomorphs are genetically predisposed to build body fat more rapidly, thus they have unique nutritional needs that may help them achieve and maintain a healthy body composition. The following food needs and justifications apply to endomorphs:

Macronutrients in Balance:

- An optimal macronutrient ratio is beneficial for endomorphs. This typically means consuming a diet rich in healthy fats, proteins, and carbohydrates in moderation. Blood sugar control and energy balance may both benefit from a diet rich in micronutrients that are in balance.

Keeping Carbohydrates Under Control:

- Endomorphs need to be very mindful of how much they consume in carbohydrates. Select complex carbohydrates like whole grains, veggies, and legumes over processed grains and refined sugars. This helps to avoid excessive fat accumulation and stabilize blood sugar levels.

Portion Control:

- Because endomorphs are more likely to store excess calories as fat, they should be mindful of the amounts they eat. Consuming fewer, better-balanced meals throughout the day may help regulate the amount of calories consumed and metabolism.

Consistent Eating Plan:

- Endomorphs, who are prone to weight gain, should pay particular attention to maintaining a regular meal schedule as it may assist regulate blood sugar levels and decrease overeating.

High-Fibre Foods:

- Rich in fiber, foods like fruits, vegetables, and whole grains help to keep hunger at bay since they are filling. They support digestive health, which is critical to overall well-being.

Lean Proteins:

- Protein helps control hunger and is essential for maintaining muscular mass. Avoid higher-fat protein substitutes and choose lean protein sources like lentils, fish, chicken, and tofu.

Healthy Fats:

- Nuts, seeds, avocados, and olive oil are all excellent sources of healthy fats. Healthy fats help with calorie management, satisfy hunger, and provide essential nutrients.

Reduced Sugar Consumption:

- Cut down on added sugars, since they may promote the formation of fat and induce blood sugar spikes and crashes. Processed food and beverages should be avoided.

Drink plenty of water:

- Both general health and metabolism depend on enough hydration. Drinking water at various times of the day may help control hunger and promote the body's natural fat-burning processes.

Regular Meals and Snacks:

- Try to include wholesome snacks in between meals and try not to skip any. This reduces the likelihood of overeating, supports stable energy levels, and helps to maintain blood sugar levels.

Less Processed Meals:

- Processed foods are sometimes heavy in calories, unhealthy fats, and sugars that are disguised. Cutting less on fast and processed foods can help you control how many calories you eat.

Personalized Approach:

- Individual nutritional needs may vary significantly, even if these general suggestions are helpful. Certain endomorphs may have specific dietary preferences or benefit from slightly different macronutrient ratios. A nutritionist or qualified dietitian with expertise in customized meal planning may be very helpful.

Patience and persistence:

- Achieving and maintaining a healthy body composition requires both patience and consistency. Remain patient and dedicated to your food plan, and be prepared to adjust as necessary based on your progress.

How to Create an Endomorph Diet Plan

Developing a diet plan tailored to your endomorph body type involves choosing specific foods that support your goals for body composition, metabolism, and overall health. Here's how to create an endomorph diet plan step-by-step:

- ***Ascertain Your Needs for Calories:*** Determine how many calories you need each day based on your age, gender, level of activity, and objectives (for example, weight reduction or muscle building). There are a lot of online calculators that may help you estimate this.

- ***Macronutrient Balance:*** Make sure your intake of macronutrients is in balance. A ratio of around 40% carbohydrates, 30% protein, and 30% healthy fats is a good place to start. You should modify these ratios according to your preferences and your body's response.

- ***Select Complex Carbohydrates:*** Give preference to complex carbohydrates over simple ones, such as whole grains (brown rice, quinoa, and whole wheat), vegetables, and legumes. These provide sustained energy and help to stabilize blood sugar levels, which reduces the production of fat.

- ***Include Lean Proteins:*** The best sources of lean protein include fish, poultry, tofu, tempeh, lean cattle or pig cuts, and lentils. Protein helps control appetite and maintain muscles.

- ***Good Fats:*** Include fatty fish (salmon, mackerel) and avocados in your diet, along with nuts, seeds, and olive oil. These fats boost satiety and provide essential nutrients.

- **Portion Control:** Pay attention to serving sizes, particularly when consuming foods rich in calories. Use a food scale and measuring cups if needed until you have a firm grasp on serving sizes.

- **Eat Meals High in Fiber:** Consume foods high in fiber, such as whole grains, fruits, and vegetables. Fiber promotes overall health, aids with digestion, and boosts satiety.

- **Manage Your Sugar Intake:** Limit the amount of processed carbohydrates and added sugars you consume. This prevents blood sugar spikes and falls, which lowers the buildup of fat.

- **Regular Meal Scheduling:** Keep up a regular eating schedule that consists of three main meals and wholesome snacks throughout the day. This helps to maintain stable blood sugar levels and control appetite.

- **Hydration:** To keep hydrated, drink plenty of water throughout the day. Sometimes hunger might be mistaken for thirst.

- **Select Foods High in Nutrients:** Make consuming meals rich in vitamins and minerals and minimal in calories a priority. Lean meats, vibrant vegetables, and leafy greens are a few examples.

- ***Meal Preparation:*** Plan your meals to ensure that wholesome options are readily accessible and to reduce the temptation to make less nourishing choices when you're hungry.

- ***Monitor Your Progress:*** Maintain a food diary to record your daily intake and see how your body responds to different meals and mealtimes.

- ***Be Flexible and Patient:*** Understand that it takes time to achieve and maintain a healthy body composition. Treat yourself with respect, and don't hesitate to adjust your diet in response to your body's response and your test findings.

Balance of Macronutrients and Control of Portion

A healthy diet must include portion control and macronutrient balance; individuals who want to reduce weight, alter their body composition, or achieve certain nutritional goals should pay particular attention to these aspects of their diet. Let's examine each of these concepts in more detail:

Control of Portion:

The regulation of the quantity of food eaten in a single dish or meal is known as portion control. It's a useful habit since it enables you to:

- Limit Calorie Intake: Eating in moderation will help you avoid overindulging and consuming too many calories, which is crucial for maintaining a healthy weight.

- Lower serving sizes promote attentive eating, when you taste your food and pay attention to signals of fullness and hunger.

- Prevent Food Waste: By making sure that just what is needed is prepared and eaten, proper portion control helps to prevent food waste.

Here are a few useful pointers regarding portion management:

- Use smaller plates and platters to organically reduce portion sizes.

- Look for information about serving sizes on food labels.

- Prepare your dinner by measuring or weighing everything in advance to get a sense of appropriate portions.

- In restaurants, be aware of portion distortion since some dishes are larger than required.

Macronutrient Balance:

Eating the right amounts of carbohydrates, proteins, and fats is part of macronutrient balancing. Every macronutrient has a specific function to fulfill in terms of your general nutrition and health:

- The body uses carbohydrates as its main energy source. For fiber, vitamins, and minerals, focus on complex carbohydrates such as whole grains, fruits, and vegetables.

- Many biological activities, including muscle upkeep and tissue repair, depend on proteins. Pick lean protein sources including beans, tofu, fish, poultry, and low-fat dairy.

- Fats: Nutrient absorption and overall health are enhanced by healthy fats, which also support brain function. As sources of good fats, include avocados, almonds, seeds, and olive oil in your diet.

- Macronutrient balance is essential since it: Encourages Satiety: You may reduce your risk of overeating by maintaining a longer sensation of fullness with a diet that is well-balanced in terms of carbohydrates, proteins, and fats.

- Lipids offer sustained energy, but carbohydrates supply energy instantly. An active lifestyle is dependent on the building and repair of tissues, which is facilitated by protein.

- Boosts Nutrient Intake: A diet rich in a range of essential nutrients will make sure your body gets what it needs for optimum functioning.

Use these procedures to determine the balance of macronutrients:

- Include foods from every nutritional group in your diet.
- Think about the dietary requirements specific to you, such as those of athletes, vegetarians, or those with certain medical conditions.
- Use nutrition apps or maintain a food diary to monitor your macronutrient intake and make sure you meet your goals.

Customization:

It is essential to adjust macronutrient ratios and portion sizes to your unique needs and objectives. A diet that is effective for one individual may not be for another. Your age, gender, degree of activity, and health conditions all play a role in determining the nutrients you need.

Optimal Nutrition Practices for Prolonged Achievement

Establishing and maintaining healthy eating habits is essential for achieving long-term gains in your overall health, fitness, and well-being. A balanced and long-lasting relationship with food may be developed with the help of various practices, even though there isn't a single, universally applicable approach to healthy eating. The following are some crucial good dietary habits for sustained success:

- ***Eat a Well-Balanced Diet:*** Try to maintain a balance between macronutrients (proteins, fats, and carbs) and micronutrients (vitamins and minerals). This guarantees that you get a wide range of essential nutrients.

- ***Portion Control:*** Be mindful of portion sizes to prevent overindulging. Use smaller dishes, plates, and utensils to help with portion control.

- ***Mindfulness in Eating:*** Take pleasure in each bite and be aware of your body's signals of hunger and fullness while you eat. Steer clear of temptations like electronics while eating.

- ***Hydration:*** To keep hydrated, drink plenty of water throughout the day. Hunger and thirst might be mistaken for one another.

- *Eat Whole Foods:* As whole, unprocessed foods, fruits, vegetables, whole grains, lean meats, and healthy fats should take precedence. These nutrient-dense meals support overall well-being.

- *High-Fibre Diet:* To improve fullness and assist with digestion, include meals high in fiber. High-fiber foods include whole grains, legumes, fruits, and vegetables.

- *Macronutrients in Balance:* Try to get the right amounts of carbohydrates, proteins, and fats in your meals. This facilitates the management of hunger and energy levels.

- *Good Fats:* You may get good fats from your diet by consuming avocados, nuts, seeds, and olive oil. Nutrient absorption and brain function both benefit from healthy fats.

- *Low-fat proteins:* Go for lean protein sources including fish, poultry, tofu, lentils, and dairy products with reduced fat content. Both general health and the upkeep of muscles need protein.

- *Limit Added Sugars:* Cut down on sugary drinks and added sugars since they might lead to energy surges and crashes.

- *Plan Your Meals and Snacks:* Make sure you have wholesome options on hand by scheduling your meals and snacks in advance. This reduces the urge to make unhealthy decisions while you're hungry.

- ***Cooking at Home:*** Since you have greater control over the ingredients and cooking methods, make meals at home whenever possible.

- ***Mindful Eating:*** Take into account the things that make you eat emotionally and try to discern between true hunger and emotional cravings.

- ***Be flexible:*** Permit yourself to sometimes indulge in meals or snacks that may not fit into your regular, healthful eating schedule. Being adaptable encourages a lasting relationship with food.

- ***Pay Attention to Your Body:*** Be aware of the signs your body sends when it is hungry and full. Eat just till you are satisfied and stop eating when you are full.

- ***Preserve Your Understanding:*** Keep up your knowledge of diet by consulting reliable sources and seeking out guidance from licensed nutritionists or dietitians as needed.

- ***Steer clear of excessive diets:*** Steer clear of excessive diets that offer immediate benefits. These may lead to health issues and are often unsustainable.

- ***Establish realistic goals:*** Establish realistic goals for your fitness and well-being. Long-term success is more likely to arise from little, gradual changes.

MEAL PLANNING AND RECIPES

30-Day Meal Plan

Day 1

- **Breakfast:** Scrambled eggs with spinach and feta cheese + 1 slice of whole-grain toast

- **Snack:** Greek yogurt with a handful of almonds

- **Lunch:** Grilled chicken salad with mixed greens, cherry tomatoes, cucumber, and a vinaigrette dressing

- **Snack:** Sliced apple with peanut butter

- **Dinner:** Baked salmon with asparagus and quinoa

Day 2

- **Breakfast:** Protein smoothie (whey protein, almond milk, berries, and spinach)

- **Snack:** Cottage cheese with pineapple chunks

- **Lunch:** Turkey breast wrap with whole-grain tortilla, avocado, lettuce, and tomato

- **Snack:** Carrot sticks with hummus

- **Dinner:** Stir-fried beef with broccoli and brown rice

Day 3

- **Breakfast:** Oatmeal with sliced banana and almond butter

- **Snack:** Hard-boiled eggs

- **Lunch:** Quinoa salad with chickpeas, red bell pepper, and feta cheese

- **Snack:** Mixed nuts

- **Dinner:** Grilled shrimp with mixed vegetables and sweet potato

Day 4

- **Breakfast:** Cottage cheese with fresh berries and a drizzle of honey

- **Snack:** Avocado toast on whole-grain bread

- **Lunch:** Chicken Caesar salad (use Greek yogurt for dressing)

- **Snack:** Sliced pear with a handful of walnuts

- **Dinner:** Baked tilapia with steamed green beans and wild rice

Day 5

- **Breakfast:** Greek yogurt with granola and mixed berries

- **Snack:** A small bag of trail mix

- **Lunch:** Baked cod with a side salad and balsamic vinaigrette

- **Snack:** Sliced cucumber with a tablespoon of tzatziki

- **Dinner:** Turkey chili with beans and a side of brown rice

Day 6

- **Breakfast:** Whole-grain toast with avocado and poached eggs

- **Snack:** A protein bar (low sugar)

- **Lunch:** Lentil soup with a side of mixed greens

- **Snack:** An orange and a handful of almonds

- **Dinner:** Grilled chicken breast with quinoa and steamed carrots

Day 7

- **Breakfast:** Protein pancakes with a handful of blueberries

- **Snack:** Greek yogurt

- **Lunch:** Tuna salad with mixed greens, cherry tomatoes, and olives

- **Snack:** Sliced bell peppers with hummus

- **Dinner:** Pork tenderloin with roasted Brussels sprouts and a small sweet potato

Day 8

- **Breakfast:** Smoothie with whey protein, spinach, banana, and almond milk

- **Snack:** Cottage cheese with raspberries

- **Lunch:** Grilled salmon salad with avocado and walnut pieces

- **Snack:** A pear

- **Dinner:** Chicken stir-fry with mixed vegetables and brown rice

Day 9

- **Breakfast:** Scrambled eggs with mushrooms and onions + 1 slice of whole-grain toast

- **Snack:** A handful of mixed nuts

- **Lunch:** Turkey and hummus wrap with whole-grain tortilla

- **Snack:** Apple slices with almond butter

- **Dinner:** Beef stew with a side of steamed broccoli

Day 10

- **Breakfast:** Chia seed pudding with almond milk and mixed berries

- **Snack:** A banana

- **Lunch:** Quinoa and black bean salad with corn, diced tomatoes, and avocado

- **Snack:** Raw vegetables with guacamole

- **Dinner:** Baked lemon garlic chicken with a side of roasted asparagus

Day 11

- **Breakfast:** Protein shake with whey protein, kale, banana, and peanut butter

- **Snack:** A hard-boiled egg

- **Lunch:** Spinach and feta stuffed chicken breast with a side salad

- **Snack:** Cottage cheese with sliced peaches

- **Dinner:** Shrimp and vegetable stir-fry over quinoa

Day 12

- **Breakfast:** Overnight oats with chia seeds, almond milk, and blueberries

- **Snack:** A small handful of walnuts

- **Lunch:** Chicken Caesar wrap with a whole-grain tortilla

- **Snack:** Sliced cucumber and cherry tomatoes with balsamic glaze

- **Dinner:** Turkey meatballs with spaghetti squash and marinara sauce

Day 13

- **Breakfast:** Green smoothie with spinach, avocado, banana, and protein powder

- **Snack:** Greek yogurt with honey and almonds

- **Lunch:** Grilled vegetable and quinoa salad with a lemon-tahini dressing

- **Snack:** An apple

- **Dinner:** Pan-seared salmon with a side of wild rice and steamed green beans

Day 14

- **Breakfast:** Egg muffins with spinach, tomatoes, and onions

- **Snack:** A protein bar

- **Lunch:** Chickpea and avocado salad

- **Snack:** A peach

- **Dinner:** Grilled steak with a side of roasted sweet potatoes and a green salad

Day 15

- **Breakfast:** Berry protein smoothie with spinach, mixed berries, whey protein, and almond milk

- **Snack:** A handful of almonds and a piece of fruit

- **Lunch:** Tuna stuffed avocado

- **Snack:** Sliced bell peppers and hummus

- **Dinner:** Lemon herb chicken with quinoa and steamed broccoli

Day 16

- **Breakfast:** Whole grain toast with almond butter and banana slices

- **Snack:** Cottage cheese with sliced strawberries

- **Lunch:** Lentil and vegetable stew

- **Snack:** A small bag of trail mix

- **Dinner:** Baked trout with a side of sautéed kale and mashed cauliflower

Day 17

- **Breakfast:** Scrambled tofu with spinach, mushrooms, and tomatoes

- **Snack:** A protein shake

- **Lunch:** Chicken and avocado salad with mixed greens, cucumber, and a vinaigrette dressing

- **Snack:** An orange

- **Dinner:** Beef and vegetable stir-fry with brown rice

Day 18

- **Breakfast:** Greek yogurt with granola and a handful of raspberries

- **Snack:** A small handful of cashews

- **Lunch:** Quinoa salad with roasted vegetables and feta cheese

- **Snack:** Sliced apple with peanut butter

- **Dinner:** Grilled pork chop with steamed green beans and sweet potato wedges

Day 19

- **Breakfast:** Smoothie bowl with whey protein, mixed berries, spinach, and a sprinkle of chia seeds

- **Snack:** Hard-boiled eggs

- **Lunch:** Turkey burger (no bun) with a side salad

- **Snack:** A handful of cherry tomatoes and mozzarella balls

- **Dinner:** Baked cod with roasted Brussels sprouts and quinoa

Day 20

- **Breakfast:** Omelet with mixed vegetables and a slice of whole-grain toast

- **Snack:** Greek yogurt with sliced almonds

- **Lunch:** Chicken and vegetable soup with a side of whole-grain bread

- **Snack:** A banana

- **Dinner:** Lamb skewers with tzatziki sauce and a Greek salad

Day 21

- **Breakfast:** Protein pancake with a handful of strawberries and a drizzle of agave syrup

- **Snack:** A small bag of trail mix

- **Lunch:** Spinach and goat cheese stuffed chicken breast with a side of roasted carrots

- **Snack:** An apple

- **Dinner:** Grilled shrimp over mixed greens with avocado, mango, and a lime vinaigrette

Day 22

- **Breakfast:** Chia seed pudding made with almond milk and topped with kiwi and coconut flakes

- **Snack:** A handful of walnuts

- **Lunch:** Grilled salmon with a side of asparagus and a quinoa salad

- **Snack:** Carrot sticks with hummus

- **Dinner:** Chicken fajitas with peppers and onions served on whole-grain tortillas

Day 23

- **Breakfast:** Avocado toast on whole-grain bread with poached eggs

- **Snack:** A protein shake

- **Lunch:** Mixed bean salad with corn, diced bell peppers, lime, and cilantro

- **Snack:** Greek yogurt with a sprinkle of cinnamon

- **Dinner:** Turkey meatloaf with a side of steamed broccoli and mashed sweet potatoes

Day 24

- **Breakfast:** Smoothie with almond milk, banana, peanut butter, and protein powder

- **Snack:** A hard-boiled egg

- **Lunch:** Sardine salad with mixed greens, olives, and a vinaigrette dressing

- **Snack:** Sliced cucumber with a tablespoon of tzatziki

- **Dinner:** Quinoa stuffed bell peppers with marinara sauce

Day 25

- **Breakfast:** Cottage cheese with pineapple and a sprinkle of chia seeds

- **Snack:** A small handful of almonds

- **Lunch:** Roasted turkey breast slices with a side of quinoa and steamed green beans

- **Snack:** An orange

- **Dinner:** Baked haddock with a side of roasted Brussels sprouts and a sweet potato

Day 26

- **Breakfast:** Protein smoothie with whey protein, almond milk, spinach, and mixed berries

- **Snack:** A banana

- **Lunch:** Chicken gyro salad with tzatziki dressing

- **Snack:** A small handful of mixed nuts

- **Dinner:** Beef stir-fry with vegetables and brown rice

Day 27

- **Breakfast:** Oatmeal with almond milk, sliced almonds, and blueberries

- **Snack:** Greek yogurt with a drizzle of honey

- **Lunch:** Baked salmon with a side salad and balsamic vinaigrette

- **Snack:** Carrot and celery sticks with hummus

- **Dinner:** Chicken parmesan with a side of spaghetti squash

Day 28

- **Breakfast:** Scrambled eggs with diced tomatoes, onions, and spinach

- **Snack:** A small bag of trail mix

- **Lunch:** Tuna salad served over mixed greens with avocado slices

- **Snack:** Sliced bell peppers

- **Dinner:** Pork tenderloin with roasted root vegetables

Day 29

- **Breakfast:** Green smoothie with spinach, avocado, protein powder, and a small apple

- **Snack:** Cottage cheese with sliced peaches

- **Lunch:** Grilled chicken breast with a kale and quinoa salad

- **Snack:** A handful of berries

- **Dinner:** Baked trout with steamed asparagus and wild rice

Day 30

- **Breakfast:** Whole-grain waffles with natural peanut butter and sliced bananas

- **Snack:** A protein bar

- **Lunch:** Quinoa and black bean stuffed peppers

- **Snack:** An apple

- **Dinner:** Lemon garlic roasted chicken with a side of brussels sprouts and a quinoa pilaf

Breakfast Recipe

Protein-Packed Spinach & Feta Omelet

- **Prep Time:** 5 minutes

  Cooking Time: 10 minutes

  Serving Size: 1

Ingredients:

- 3 large eggs

- 1 cup fresh spinach, chopped

- 1/4 cup feta cheese, crumbled

- 1/4 cup red bell pepper, diced

- Salt and pepper to taste

- 1 tsp olive oil

Instructions:

1. In a bowl, whisk the eggs until well beaten. Stir in the spinach, feta cheese, red bell pepper, salt, and pepper.

2. Heat olive oil in a non-stick skillet over medium heat.

3. Pour the egg mixture into the skillet. Cook for 4-5 minutes until the edges start to lift from the pan.

4. Carefully flip the omelet and cook for an additional 3-4 minutes or until the eggs are set and the feta is slightly melted.

5. Serve immediately.

Nutritional Information:

- Calories: 320

- Protein: 24g

- Carbohydrates: 6g

- Fat: 22g

- Fiber: 1g

- Sodium: 710mg

Almond Butter & Banana Protein Smoothie

- **Prep Time:** 5 minutes
  Cooking Time: 0 minutes
  Serving Size: 1

Ingredients:

- 1 large banana

- 2 tablespoons almond butter

- 1 cup unsweetened almond milk

- 1 scoop vanilla protein powder

- Ice cubes (optional)

Instructions:

1. Place all ingredients in a blender.

2. Blend on high until smooth.

3. Pour into a glass and serve immediately.

Nutritional Information:

- Calories: 380

- Protein: 25g

- Carbohydrates: 30g

- Fat: 18g

- Fiber: 5g

- Sodium: 220mg

Quinoa & Berry Breakfast Bowl

- **Prep Time:** 5 minutes
  Cooking Time: 15 minutes
  Serving Size: 1

Ingredients:

- 1/2 cup quinoa, rinsed

- 1 cup water

- 1/2 cup mixed berries (strawberries, blueberries, raspberries)

- 1 tablespoon chia seeds

- 1 tablespoon honey

- 1/4 cup unsweetened almond milk

Instructions:

1. In a small saucepan, bring quinoa and water to a boil. Reduce heat to low, cover, and simmer for 15 minutes or until water is absorbed.

2. Remove from heat and let it stand covered for 5 minutes. Fluff with a fork.

3. Transfer cooked quinoa to a bowl. Top with mixed berries, chia seeds, and honey.

4. Pour almond milk over the bowl and serve.

Nutritional Information:

- Calories: 330

- Protein: 12g

- Carbohydrates: 55g

- Fat: 7g

- Fiber: 8g

- Sodium: 30mg

Avocado Egg Toast

- **Prep Time:** 5 minutes

  Cooking Time: 5 minutes

  Serving Size: 1

Ingredients:

- 1 slice of whole-grain bread

- 1/2 ripe avocado

- 1 egg

- Salt and pepper to taste

- 1 tsp olive oil

Instructions:

1. Toast the whole-grain bread to your liking.

2. In a skillet, heat olive oil over medium heat and carefully crack the egg into the skillet. Cook to your preference (e.g., sunny-side up, over-easy).

3. Mash the avocado and spread it on the toasted bread.

4. Place the cooked egg over the avocado. Season with salt and pepper.

5. Serve immediately.

Nutritional Information:

- Calories: 300

- Protein: 12g

- Carbohydrates: 18g

- Fat: 20g

- Fiber: 7g

- Sodium: 200mg

Greek Yogurt with Mixed Nuts and Honey

- **Prep Time:** 5 minutes
  Cooking Time: 0 minutes
  Serving Size: 1

Ingredients:

- 1 cup Greek yogurt

- 1/4 cup mixed nuts (almonds, walnuts, pistachios), chopped

- 1 tablespoon honey

Instructions:

1. In a bowl, combine Greek yogurt and chopped nuts.

2. Drizzle honey over the top.

3. Serve immediately.

Nutritional Information:

- Calories: 320

- Protein: 20g

- Carbohydrates: 24g

- Fat: 16g

- Fiber: 2g

- Sodium: 60mg

Cottage Cheese and Pineapple Bowl

- **Prep Time:** 5 minutes
  Cooking Time: 0 minutes
  Serving Size: 1

Ingredients:

- 1 cup cottage cheese

- 1/2 cup pineapple chunks

- 1 tablespoon chia seeds

Instructions:

1. In a bowl, combine cottage cheese and pineapple chunks.

2. Sprinkle chia seeds on top.

3. Serve immediately.

Nutritional Information:

- Calories: 280

- Protein: 28g

- Carbohydrates: 25g

- Fat: 8g

- Fiber: 4g

- Sodium: 500mg

Oatmeal with Almond Milk and Blueberries

- **Prep Time:** 5 minutes
  Cooking Time: 10 minutes
  Serving Size: 1

Ingredients:

- 1/2 cup rolled oats

- 1 cup unsweetened almond milk

- 1/2 cup blueberries

- 1 tablespoon almond slices

- 1 teaspoon honey

Instructions:

1. In a small saucepan, bring almond milk to a boil.

2. Add rolled oats and reduce heat to simmer. Cook for 10 minutes, stirring occasionally, until oats are soft and creamy.

3. Transfer the oatmeal to a bowl. Top with blueberries, almond slices, and a drizzle of honey.

4. Serve immediately.

Nutritional Information:

- Calories: 290

- Protein: 8g

- Carbohydrates: 45g

- Fat: 9g

- Fiber: 7g

- Sodium: 80mg

Turkey and Spinach Breakfast Burritos

- **Prep Time:** 10 minutes

  Cooking Time: 10 minutes

  Serving Size: 2 burritos

Ingredients:

- 2 whole wheat tortillas

- 4 egg whites

- 1/2 cup cooked turkey breast, chopped

- 1 cup fresh spinach

- 1/4 cup shredded low-fat cheese

- Salt and pepper to taste

- 1 tsp olive oil

Instructions:

1. Heat olive oil in a non-stick skillet over medium heat. Add egg whites and scramble until nearly set.

2. Add chopped turkey and spinach to the skillet. Cook until spinach is wilted and turkey is heated through.

3. Warm tortillas according to package instructions.

4. Divide the egg mixture between the tortillas. Top with shredded cheese.

5. Roll up burritos, folding in the sides. Serve immediately.

Nutritional Information (per burrito):

- Calories: 300

- Protein: 28g

- Carbohydrates: 22g

- Fat: 10g

- Fiber: 3g

- Sodium: 540mg

Chia Seed Pudding with Coconut Milk

- **Prep Time:** 5 minutes (plus overnight soaking)
  Cooking Time: 0 minutes
  Serving Size: 1

Ingredients:

- 1/4 cup chia seeds

- 1 cup unsweetened coconut milk

- 1 tablespoon maple syrup

- 1/2 teaspoon vanilla extract

- Fresh berries for topping

Instructions:

1. In a bowl, mix chia seeds, coconut milk, maple syrup, and vanilla extract.

2. Cover and refrigerate overnight or at least 6 hours until it achieves a pudding-like consistency.

3. Serve topped with fresh berries.

Nutritional Information:

- Calories: 350

- Protein: 5g

- Carbohydrates: 35g

- Fat: 22g

- Fiber: 10g

- Sodium: 50mg

Savory Mushroom and Spinach Breakfast Muffins

- **Prep Time:** 15 minutes
  Cooking Time: 20 minutes
  Serving Size: 6 muffins

Ingredients:

- 6 large eggs

- 1/2 cup diced mushrooms

- 1/2 cup chopped spinach

- 1/4 cup diced onions

- 1/4 cup grated low-fat cheese

- Salt and pepper to taste

- 1 tsp olive oil

Instructions:

1. Preheat the oven to 350°F (175°C). Grease a 6-cup muffin tin with olive oil.

2. In a skillet, sauté mushrooms and onions in olive oil until softened. Add spinach and cook until wilted. Set aside to cool.

3. In a large bowl, whisk the eggs. Stir in the cooked vegetables and cheese. Season with salt and pepper.

4. Divide the mixture evenly among the muffin cups.

5. Bake for 20 minutes, or until muffins are set and lightly golden on top.

6. Allow to cool for a few minutes before removing from the tin. Serve warm.

Nutritional Information (per muffin):

- Calories: 100

- Protein: 9g

- Carbohydrates: 2g

- Fat: 6g

- Fiber: 0.5g

- Sodium: 200mg

Lunch Recipe

Grilled Chicken Salad with Avocado Dressing

- **Prep Time:** 15 minutes
  Cooking Time: 10 minutes
  Serving Size: 2

Ingredients:

- 2 boneless, skinless chicken breasts

- 4 cups mixed greens (spinach, arugula, romaine)

- 1/2 cup cherry tomatoes, halved

- 1/4 cup cucumber, sliced

- 1/4 cup red onion, thinly sliced

- 1 ripe avocado

- 2 tablespoons Greek yogurt

- 1 tablespoon lime juice

- Salt and pepper to taste

- 1 tablespoon olive oil

Instructions:

1. Season chicken breasts with salt and pepper. Grill over medium heat for 5 minutes on each side, or until cooked through. Let it rest before slicing.

2. In a blender, combine avocado, Greek yogurt, lime juice, salt, and pepper. Blend until smooth for the dressing.

3. In a large bowl, toss mixed greens, cherry tomatoes, cucumber, and red onion.

4. Add sliced chicken to the salad and drizzle with avocado dressing.

5. Serve immediately.

Nutritional Information:

- Calories: 350

- Protein: 38g

- Carbohydrates: 18g

- Fat: 16g

- Fiber: 7g

- Sodium: 220mg

Quinoa and Black Bean Bowl

- **Prep Time:** 10 minutes
  Cooking Time: 20 minutes
  Serving Size: 2

Ingredients:

- 1 cup quinoa

- 2 cups water

- 1 can (15 oz) black beans, drained and rinsed

- 1/2 cup corn kernels

- 1/2 red bell pepper, diced

- 1/4 cup fresh cilantro, chopped

- 2 tablespoons lime juice

- Salt and pepper to taste

- 1 avocado, sliced

Instructions:

1. Rinse quinoa under cold water. In a saucepan, bring quinoa and water to a boil. Reduce heat, cover, and simmer for 15 minutes or until water is absorbed.

2. Fluff quinoa with a fork and let it cool.

3. In a large bowl, mix cooled quinoa, black beans, corn, red bell pepper, and cilantro.

4. Dress with lime juice, salt, and pepper. Toss well.

5. Serve in bowls topped with sliced avocado.

Nutritional Information:

- Calories: 480

- Protein: 18g

- Carbohydrates: 70g

- Fat: 15g

- Fiber: 15g

- Sodium: 30mg

Turkey and Vegetable Wrap

- **Prep Time:** 10 minutes
  Cooking Time: 0 minutes
  Serving Size: 2 wraps

Ingredients:

- 2 whole wheat tortillas
- 4 slices of turkey breast
- 1/2 cup mixed greens
- 1/4 cup shredded carrots
- 1/4 cup cucumber, sliced
- 2 tablespoons hummus
- Salt and pepper to taste

Instructions:

1. Lay out the tortillas and spread 1 tablespoon of hummus on each.

2. Place two slices of turkey breast on each tortilla.

3. Add mixed greens, shredded carrots, and cucumber slices over the turkey.

4. Season with salt and pepper.

5. Roll up the tortillas tightly, cut in half, and serve.

Nutritional Information:

- Calories: 260
- Protein: 20g

- Carbohydrates: 35g

- Fat: 7g

- Fiber: 5g

- Sodium: 690mg

Tuna Salad Stuffed Avocado

- **Prep Time:** 10 minutes
  Cooking Time: 0 minutes
  Serving Size: 2

Ingredients:

- 1 can (5 oz) tuna in water, drained

- 1/4 cup Greek yogurt

- 1/4 cup red onion, finely chopped

- 1/4 cup celery, finely chopped

- Salt and pepper to taste

- 2 ripe avocados, halved and pitted

- 1 tablespoon lemon juice

Instructions:

1. In a bowl, mix tuna, Greek yogurt, red onion, celery, salt, and pepper.

2. Drizzle lemon juice over avocado halves to prevent browning.

3. Scoop the tuna mixture into the avocado halves.

4. Serve immediately.

Nutritional Information:

- Calories: 370

- Protein: 23g

- Carbohydrates: 17g

- Fat: 25g

- Fiber: 11g

- Sodium: 320mg

Spicy Chickpea and Quinoa Bowl

- **Prep Time:** 15 minutes
  Cooking Time: 20 minutes
  Serving Size: 2

Ingredients:

- 1 cup quinoa

- 2 cups vegetable broth

- 1 can (15 oz) chickpeas, drained, rinsed, and dried

- 1 teaspoon chili powder

- 1/2 teaspoon cumin

- 1/2 cup cherry tomatoes, halved

- 1/2 cucumber, diced

- 1/4 cup red onion, finely chopped

- 2 tablespoons olive oil

- Salt and pepper to taste

- 1 avocado, sliced

- 2 tablespoons lemon juice

Instructions:

1. Cook quinoa in vegetable broth according to package instructions. Set aside to cool.

2. Toss chickpeas with chili powder, cumin, salt, and pepper.

3. Heat olive oil in a pan over medium heat. Add seasoned chickpeas and cook until crispy, about 10 minutes.

4. In a bowl, mix cooled quinoa, cherry tomatoes, cucumber, and red onion.

5. Divide the quinoa mixture into bowls. Top with crispy chickpeas and sliced avocado.

6. Drizzle with lemon juice and serve.

Nutritional Information:

- Calories: 540

- Protein: 18g

- Carbohydrates: 70g

- Fat: 23g

- Fiber: 15g

- Sodium: 300mg

Lemon Herb Grilled Salmon

- **Prep Time:** 15 minutes (plus marinating time)
  Cooking Time: 10 minutes
  Serving Size: 2

Ingredients:

- 2 salmon fillets (6 oz each)

- 2 tablespoons olive oil

- 1 tablespoon lemon juice

- 1 teaspoon dried herbs (thyme, oregano, basil)

- Salt and pepper to taste

- 1 lemon, sliced for garnish

- 1/2 pound asparagus, trimmed

Instructions:

1. Marinate salmon with olive oil, lemon juice, dried herbs, salt, and pepper for at least 30 minutes in the refrigerator.

2. Preheat the grill to medium-high heat.

3. Grill salmon for 5 minutes per side, or until desired doneness.

4. Grill asparagus alongside salmon until tender and charred about 5 minutes.

5. Serve salmon and asparagus garnished with lemon slices.

Nutritional Information:

- Calories: 420

- Protein: 35g

- Carbohydrates: 6g

- Fat: 30g

- Fiber: 3g

- Sodium: 75mg

Beef and Broccoli Stir-Fry

- **Prep Time:** 15 minutes
  Cooking Time: 10 minutes
  Serving Size: 2

Ingredients:

- 1/2 pound lean beef, thinly sliced

- 2 cups broccoli florets

- 1 tablespoon olive oil

- 2 cloves garlic, minced

- 1/4 cup soy sauce (low sodium)

- 1 tablespoon ginger, grated

- 1 tablespoon honey

- 1 teaspoon cornstarch dissolved in 2 tablespoons water

Instructions:

1. Heat olive oil in a large pan over medium-high heat. Add garlic and ginger, sautéing until fragrant.

2. Add beef and cook until browned.

3. Add broccoli and cook for another 3-4 minutes until tender.

4. Mix soy sauce, honey, and cornstarch mixture. Add to the pan, stirring until the sauce thickens.

5. Serve immediately.

Nutritional Information:

- Calories: 300

- Protein: 26g

- Carbohydrates: 18g

- Fat: 14g

- Fiber: 3g

- Sodium: 660mg

Mediterranean Chickpea Salad

- **Prep Time:** 15 minutes
  Cooking Time: 0 minutes
  Serving Size: 2

Ingredients:

- 1 can (15 oz) chickpeas, drained and rinsed

- 1 cup cherry tomatoes, halved

- 1 cucumber, diced

- 1/4 cup red onion, finely chopped

- 1/4 cup kalamata olives, halved

- 1/4 cup feta cheese, crumbled

- 2 tablespoons olive oil

- 1 tablespoon lemon juice

- Salt and pepper to taste

- 1 teaspoon dried oregano

Instructions:

1. In a large bowl, combine chickpeas, cherry tomatoes, cucumber, red onion, kalamata olives, and feta cheese.

2. Dress with olive oil, lemon juice, salt, pepper, and dried oregano. Toss well.

3. Chill for at least 30 minutes before serving to enhance flavors.

Nutritional Information:

- Calories: 350

- Protein: 12g

- Carbohydrates: 35g

- Fat: 18g

- Fiber: 10g

- Sodium: 700mg

Sweet Potato and Black Bean Burritos

- **Prep Time:** 20 minutes

  Cooking Time: 25 minutes

  Serving Size: 4 burritos

Ingredients:

- 2 medium sweet potatoes, peeled and diced

- 1 can (15 oz) black beans, drained and rinsed

- 1 teaspoon cumin

- 1/2 teaspoon chili powder

- 1/4 cup cilantro, chopped

- 4 whole wheat tortillas

- 1/2 cup grated low-fat cheese

- 1 avocado, sliced

- Salt and pepper to taste

Instructions:

1. Preheat the oven to 400°F (200°C). Toss sweet potatoes with cumin, chili powder, salt, and pepper. Roast for 20 minutes, or until tender.

2. Warm tortillas according to package instructions.

3. Divide roasted sweet potatoes, black beans, cilantro, cheese, and avocado slices among the tortillas.

4. Roll up burritos, folding in the sides. Serve warm.

Nutritional Information:

- Calories: 450

- Protein: 14g

- Carbohydrates: 65g

- Fat: 15g

- Fiber: 15g

- Sodium: 550mg

Cauliflower Rice Stir-Fry

- **Prep Time:** 10 minutes
  Cooking Time: 15 minutes
  Serving Size: 2

Ingredients:

- 1 head cauliflower, grated into 'rice'

- 1 tablespoon sesame oil

- 1/2 cup peas

- 1/2 cup carrots, diced

- 2 eggs, beaten

- 2 tablespoons soy sauce (low sodium)

- 1 tablespoon ginger, grated

- 2 green onions, chopped

Instructions:

1. Heat sesame oil in a large skillet over medium heat. Add peas and carrots; cook until soft.

2. Push vegetables to the side, add eggs to the skillet, and scramble.

3. Add cauliflower rice, soy sauce, and ginger. Cook, stirring frequently, for 5-7 minutes.

4. Garnish with green onions before serving.

Nutritional Information:

- Calories: 220

- Protein: 12g

- Carbohydrates: 22g

- Fat: 10g

- Fiber: 6g

- Sodium: 630mg

Dinner Recipe

Baked Salmon with Dill and Lemon

- **Prep Time:** 10 minutes
  Cooking Time: 20 minutes
  Serving Size: 2

Ingredients:

- 2 salmon fillets (6 oz each)

- 1 tablespoon olive oil

- 1 lemon, sliced

- 2 teaspoons fresh dill, chopped

- Salt and pepper to taste

Instructions:

1. Preheat your oven to 400°F (200°C). Line a baking sheet with parchment paper.

2. Place the salmon fillets on the baking sheet. Drizzle with olive oil and season with salt and pepper.

3. Top each fillet with lemon slices and sprinkle with dill.

4. Bake for 20 minutes or until salmon flakes easily with a fork.

5. Serve immediately, garnished with additional fresh dill
   if desired.

Nutritional Information:

- Calories: 280

- Protein: 34g

- Carbohydrates: 0g

- Fat: 16g

- Fiber: 0g

- Sodium: 75mg

Zucchini Noodles with Turkey Meatballs

- **Prep Time:** 20 minutes
  Cooking Time: 30 minutes
  Serving Size: 2

Ingredients:

- 2 large zucchinis

- 1/2 pound ground turkey

- 1/4 cup breadcrumbs

- 1 egg

- 1 teaspoon garlic powder

- 1 teaspoon onion powder

- 1 cup marinara sauce, low-sodium

- Salt and pepper to taste

- 1 tablespoon olive oil

Instructions:

1. Spiralize the zucchini to create noodles. Set aside.

2. In a bowl, mix ground turkey, breadcrumbs, egg, garlic powder, onion powder, salt, and pepper. Form into small meatballs.

3. Heat olive oil in a pan over medium heat. Cook meatballs until browned and cooked through about 10 minutes.

4. Add marinara sauce to the pan and simmer for another 10 minutes.

5. In a separate pan, sauté zucchini noodles in a bit of olive oil for 2-3 minutes, until just tender.

6. Serve meatballs and sauce over the zucchini noodles.

Nutritional Information:

- Calories: 400

- Protein: 36g

- Carbohydrates: 18g

- Fat: 20g

- Fiber: 4g

- Sodium: 320mg

Grilled Vegetable Quinoa Salad

- **Prep Time:** 15 minutes
  Cooking Time: 15 minutes
  Serving Size: 2

Ingredients:

- 1 cup quinoa, cooked

- 1 zucchini, sliced

- 1 bell pepper, sliced

- 1/2 red onion, sliced

- 2 tablespoons olive oil

- 1 tablespoon balsamic vinegar

- Salt and pepper to taste

- 1/4 cup feta cheese, crumbled

- 2 tablespoons fresh parsley, chopped

Instructions:

1. Preheat the grill to medium-high heat.

2. Toss zucchini, bell pepper, and red onion with 1 tablespoon olive oil, salt, and pepper.

3. Grill vegetables until charred and tender, about 5-7 minutes, turning occasionally.

4. In a large bowl, combine cooked quinoa, grilled vegetables, remaining olive oil, balsamic vinegar, feta cheese, and parsley. Toss gently.

5. Serve warm or at room temperature.

Nutritional Information:

- Calories: 370

- Protein: 12g

- Carbohydrates: 45g

- Fat: 16g

- Fiber: 6g

- Sodium: 200mg

Slow Cooker Chicken Cacciatore

- **Prep Time:** 15 minutes

  Cooking Time: 4 hours on high

  Serving Size: 2

Ingredients:

- 2 chicken breasts, boneless and skinless

- 1 can (14 oz) diced tomatoes

- 1 bell pepper, sliced

- 1/2 red onion, sliced

- 2 cloves garlic, minced

- 1 teaspoon dried oregano

- 1 teaspoon dried basil

- Salt and pepper to taste

Instructions:

1. Place chicken breasts at the bottom of the slow cooker.

2. Top with diced tomatoes, bell pepper, onion, garlic, oregano, basil, salt, and pepper.

3. Cover and cook on high for 4 hours or until chicken is tender.

4. Shred the chicken in the sauce and mix well.

5. Serve hot, garnished with fresh basil if desired.

Nutritional Information:

- Calories: 260

- Protein: 36g

- Carbohydrates: 15g

- Fat: 4g

- Fiber: 3g

- Sodium: 320mg

Spicy Shrimp and Cauliflower Rice Bowl

- **Prep Time:** 15 minutes
  Cooking Time: 10 minutes
  Serving Size: 2

Ingredients:

- 1 head cauliflower, grated into 'rice'

- 1 pound shrimp, peeled and deveined

- 1 tablespoon olive oil

- 1 teaspoon chili powder

- 1/2 teaspoon garlic powder

- 1/2 teaspoon paprika

- Salt and pepper to taste

- 1 avocado, sliced

- 1 lime, cut into wedges

Instructions:

1. Heat olive oil in a large skillet over medium heat. Add cauliflower rice and cook for 5-7 minutes, until tender. Remove from skillet and set aside.

2. In the same skillet, add shrimp, chili powder, garlic powder, paprika, salt, and pepper. Cook until shrimp are pink and cooked through about 3-5 minutes.

3. Divide cauliflower rice between bowls. Top with spicy shrimp, avocado slices, and a lime wedge.

4. Serve immediately.

Nutritional Information:

- Calories: 390

- Protein: 48g

- Carbohydrates: 18g

- Fat: 16g

- Fiber: 7g

- Sodium: 350mg

Turkey and Spinach Stuffed Peppers

- **Prep Time:** 20 minutes

  Cooking Time: 25 minutes

  Serving Size: 2

Ingredients:

- 2 bell peppers, halved and deseeded

- 1/2 pound ground turkey

- 2 cups spinach, chopped

- 1/4 cup quinoa, cooked

- 1/2 cup marinara sauce, low sodium

- 1/4 cup mozzarella cheese, shredded

- Salt and pepper to taste

Instructions:

1. Preheat oven to 375°F (190°C).

2. In a skillet, cook ground turkey over medium heat until browned. Drain excess fat.

3. Stir in spinach and cook until wilted. Add cooked quinoa and marinara sauce. Season with salt and pepper.

4. Fill each bell pepper half with the turkey mixture. Top with shredded mozzarella.

5. Place stuffed peppers in a baking dish. Bake for 25 minutes, or until peppers are tender and cheese is melted.

6. Serve hot.

Nutritional Information:

- Calories: 320

- Protein: 28g

- Carbohydrates: 22g

- Fat: 14g

- Fiber: 5g

- Sodium: 400mg

Lemon Garlic Tilapia

- **Prep Time:** 10 minutes
  Cooking Time: 12 minutes
  Serving Size: 2

Ingredients:

- 2 tilapia fillets

- 2 tablespoons olive oil

- 2 cloves garlic, minced

- 1 lemon, juiced and zested

- Salt and pepper to taste

- Fresh parsley, chopped (for garnish)

Instructions:

1. Preheat oven to 400°F (200°C). Line a baking sheet with parchment paper.

2. In a small bowl, mix olive oil, garlic, lemon juice, lemon zest, salt, and pepper.

3. Place tilapia fillets on the prepared baking sheet. Drizzle with the lemon garlic mixture.

4. Bake for 10-12 minutes or until fish flakes easily with a fork.

5. Garnish with fresh parsley before serving.

Nutritional Information:

- Calories: 220

- Protein: 34g

- Carbohydrates: 2g

- Fat: 8g

- Fiber: 0g

- Sodium: 65mg

Eggplant and Chickpea Curry

- **Prep Time:** 15 minutes
  Cooking Time: 30 minutes
  Serving Size: 2

Ingredients:

- 1 large eggplant, cubed

- 1 can (15 oz) chickpeas, drained and rinsed

- 1 can (14 oz) diced tomatoes

- 1 onion, diced

- 2 cloves garlic, minced

- 1 tablespoon curry powder

- 1 teaspoon cumin

- 1/2 teaspoon turmeric

- 1/2 cup coconut milk

- Salt and pepper to taste

- 1 tablespoon olive oil

Instructions:

1. Heat olive oil in a large skillet over medium heat. Add onion and garlic, and cook until softened.

2. Add curry powder, cumin, and turmeric, stirring for 1 minute until fragrant.

3. Add eggplant, chickpeas, and diced tomatoes. Season with salt and pepper.

4. Cover and simmer for 20 minutes, or until eggplant is tender.

5. Stir in coconut milk and cook for another 10 minutes.

6. Serve hot, garnished with fresh cilantro if desired.

Nutritional Information:

- Calories: 380

- Protein: 12g

- Carbohydrates: 45g

- Fat: 18g

- Fiber: 13g

- Sodium: 320mg

Pork Tenderloin with Roasted Vegetables

- **Prep Time:** 15 minutes

  Cooking Time: 25 minutes

  Serving Size: 2

Ingredients:

- 1 pork tenderloin (about 1 pound)

- 1 sweet potato, cubed

- 1 bell pepper, cubed

- 1 zucchini, cubed

- 2 tablespoons olive oil

- 1 teaspoon rosemary

- Salt and pepper to taste

Instructions:

1. Preheat oven to 425°F (220°C). Line a large baking sheet with parchment paper.

2. Toss sweet potato, bell pepper, and zucchini with olive oil, rosemary, salt, and pepper. Spread evenly on the baking sheet.

3. Place the pork tenderloin in the center of the baking sheet, surrounded by the vegetables.

4. Roast for 25 minutes, or until the pork reaches an internal temperature of 145°F (63°C) and the vegetables are tender.

5. Let the pork rest for 5 minutes before slicing. Serve with roasted vegetables.

Nutritional Information:

- Calories: 420

- Protein: 36g

- Carbohydrates: 32g

- Fat: 18g

- Fiber: 5g

- Sodium: 110mg

Balsamic Glazed Chicken and Roasted Brussels Sprouts

- **Prep Time:** 15 minutes
  Cooking Time: 25 minutes
  Serving Size: 2

Ingredients:

- 2 chicken breasts

- 2 cups Brussels sprouts, halved

- 2 tablespoons olive oil

- 1/4 cup balsamic vinegar

- 1 tablespoon honey

- Salt and pepper to taste

- 1 garlic clove, minced

Instructions:

1. Preheat oven to 400°F (200°C). Line a baking sheet with parchment paper.

2. Toss Brussels sprouts with 1 tablespoon olive oil, salt, and pepper. Spread on half of the baking sheet.

3. In a small bowl, whisk together balsamic vinegar, honey, and garlic.

4. Place chicken breasts on the other half of the baking sheet. Season with salt and pepper. Brush with half of the balsamic mixture.

5. Bake for 20 minutes. Then, brush the chicken with the remaining balsamic mixture and bake for another 5 minutes, or until the chicken is cooked through and Brussels sprouts are caramelized.

6. Serve immediately.

Nutritional Information:

- Calories: 350

- Protein: 32g

- Carbohydrates: 22g

- Fat: 16g

- Fiber: 4g

- Sodium: 200mg

Snack Recipes

Almond Butter and Banana Rice Cakes

- **Prep Time:** 5 minutes
  Cooking Time: 0 minutes
  Serving Size: 1

Ingredients:

- 2 plain rice cakes

- 2 tablespoons almond butter

- 1 banana, sliced

- A sprinkle of cinnamon (optional)

Instructions:

1. Spread 1 tablespoon of almond butter evenly over each rice cake.

2. Arrange banana slices on top of the almond butter on each rice cake.

3. Sprinkle a dash of cinnamon over the banana slices for added flavor, if desired.

4. Serve immediately for a crunchy, sweet, and satisfying snack.

Nutritional Information:

- Calories: 280

- Protein: 7g

- Carbohydrates: 40g

- Fat: 12g

- Fiber: 5g

- Sodium: 100mg

Greek Yogurt with Mixed Berries and Nuts

- **Prep Time:** 5 minutes
  Cooking Time: 0 minutes
  Serving Size: 1

Ingredients:

- 1 cup plain Greek yogurt

- 1/2 cup mixed berries (strawberries, blueberries, raspberries)

- 1/4 cup mixed nuts (almonds, walnuts, pecans), chopped

- 1 tablespoon honey

Instructions:

1. In a bowl, add the Greek yogurt.

2. Top the yogurt with mixed berries and chopped nuts.

3. Drizzle honey over the top for a touch of sweetness.

4. Mix lightly before eating or enjoy the layers as is for a protein-rich, antioxidant-packed snack.

Nutritional Information:

- Calories: 320

- Protein: 25g

- Carbohydrates: 35g

- Fat: 12g

- Fiber: 5g

- Sodium: 60mg

Avocado and Tomato on Whole-Grain Toast

- **Prep Time:** 5 minutes

  Cooking Time: 2 minutes (to toast the bread)

  Serving Size: 1

Ingredients:

- 1 slice of whole-grain bread

- 1/2 ripe avocado

- 1 small tomato, sliced

- Salt and pepper to taste

- Red pepper flakes (optional)

Instructions:

1. Toast the whole-grain bread to your liking.

2. Mash the avocado and spread it evenly over the toasted bread.

3. Arrange tomato slices on top of the avocado.

4. Season with salt, pepper, and red pepper flakes for a little extra kick, if desired.

5. Serve immediately for a creamy, savory, and heart-healthy snack.

Nutritional Information:

- Calories: 220

- Protein: 6g

- Carbohydrates: 27g

- Fat: 11g

- Fiber: 9g

- Sodium: 200mg

Cottage Cheese and Pineapple Bowl

- **Prep Time:** 5 minutes
  Cooking Time: 0 minutes
  Serving Size: 1

Ingredients:

- 1 cup low-fat cottage cheese

- 1/2 cup pineapple chunks, fresh or canned in juice

- A sprinkle of chia seeds (optional)

Instructions:

1. In a bowl, combine the cottage cheese and pineapple chunks.

2. Sprinkle chia seeds over the top for added fiber and omega-3 fatty acids, if desired.

3. Enjoy this sweet and creamy snack that balances protein with the natural sugars of the fruit for sustained energy.

Nutritional Information:

- Calories: 200

- Protein: 28g

- Carbohydrates: 20g

- Fat: 2g

- Fiber: 2g

- Sodium: 500mg

Almond Butter Celery Sticks

- **Prep Time:** 5 minutes
  Cooking Time: 0 minutes
  Serving Size: 2 servings

Ingredients:

- 4 celery stalks, washed and cut into 3-inch pieces

- 2 tablespoons almond butter

- 1 tablespoon raisins or dried cranberries

Instructions:

1. Spread almond butter evenly inside the celery stalk pieces.

2. Sprinkle raisins or dried cranberries over the almond butter.

3. Serve as a crunchy and satisfying snack.

Nutritional Information:

- Calories: 150 per serving

- Protein: 4g

- Carbohydrates: 12g

- Fat: 10g

- Fiber: 3g

- Sodium: 150mg

Zucchini Chips with Avocado Yogurt Dip

- **Prep Time:** 15 minutes
  Cooking Time: 2 hours
  Serving Size: 4 servings

Ingredients for Zucchini Chips:

- 2 large zucchinis, thinly sliced

- 1 tablespoon olive oil

- Salt and pepper, to taste

Ingredients for Avocado Yogurt Dip:

- 1 ripe avocado

- 1/2 cup plain Greek yogurt

- 1 tablespoon lime juice

- 1 clove garlic, minced

- Salt and pepper, to taste

Instructions:

1. Preheat your oven to 225°F (105°C). Line a baking sheet with parchment paper.

2. In a bowl, toss the zucchini slices with olive oil, salt, and pepper until evenly coated.

3. Arrange the zucchini slices in a single layer on the baking sheet. Bake for 1.5 to 2 hours, flipping halfway through, until crisp and golden.

4. While the zucchini chips are baking, prepare the dip. In a bowl, mash the avocado. Mix in the Greek yogurt, lime juice, garlic, salt, and pepper until smooth and creamy.

5. Once the zucchini chips are done, let them cool before serving with the avocado yogurt dip.

Nutritional Information:

- Calories: 120 per serving

- Protein: 4g

- Carbohydrates: 8g

- Fat: 9g

- Fiber: 3g

- Sodium: 75mg

Hummus and Veggie Sticks

- **Prep Time:** 10 minutes
  Cooking Time: 0 minutes
  Serving Size: 2 servings

Ingredients:

- 1/2 cup hummus

- 1 carrot, peeled and cut into sticks

- 1 cucumber, cut into sticks

- 1 bell pepper, sliced

Instructions:

1. Prepare the vegetables by washing, peeling (if necessary), and cutting them into stick shapes.

2. Serve the hummus in a small bowl surrounded by the vegetable sticks for dipping.

3. Enjoy a refreshing and nutritious snack that's perfect for a quick energy boost.

Nutritional Information (per serving):

- Calories: 180

- Protein: 6g

- Carbohydrates: 20g

- Fat: 9g

- Fiber: 5g

- Sodium: 300mg

Cucumber Avocado Rolls

- **Prep Time:** 15 minutes
  Cooking Time: 0 minutes
  Serving Size: Makes 12 rolls

Ingredients:

- 1 large cucumber

- 1 ripe avocado

- 1/4 cup finely diced red bell pepper

- 1 tablespoon lime juice

- 1/4 teaspoon salt

- 1 tablespoon chopped cilantro

- 1/4 teaspoon chili flakes (optional)

Instructions:

1. Using a vegetable peeler or mandoline, slice the cucumber into long, thin strips.

2. In a bowl, mash the avocado and mix in lime juice, salt, diced bell pepper, cilantro, and chili flakes until well combined.

3. Lay a cucumber strip flat on a cutting board, and at one end, place a spoonful of the avocado mixture.

4. Carefully roll the cucumber around the filling, and place the roll seam-side down on a serving plate. Repeat with the remaining cucumber strips and filling.

5. Serve immediately or chill for 30 minutes before serving for a firmer texture.

Nutritional Information (per roll):

- Calories: 45

- Protein: 1g

- Carbohydrates: 3g

- Fat: 3.5g

- Fiber: 1.5g

- Sodium: 50mg

Almond Butter and Banana Open Sandwich

- **Prep Time:** 5 minutes
  Cooking Time: 0 minutes
  Serving Size: 1 sandwich

Ingredients:

- 1 slice whole grain bread, toasted

- 2 tablespoons almond butter

- 1/2 banana, sliced

- 1/4 teaspoon cinnamon

Instructions:

1. Spread the almond butter evenly over the toasted slice of whole-grain bread.

2. Arrange the banana slices on top of the almond butter.

3. Sprinkle cinnamon over the banana slices.

4. Serve immediately for a quick and nutritious snack.

Nutritional Information:

- Calories: 280

- Protein: 8g

- Carbohydrates: 30g

- Fat: 16g

- Fiber: 5g

- Sodium: 150mg

Cottage Cheese and Cherry Tomatoes

- **Prep Time:** 5 minutes
  Cooking Time: 0 minutes
  Serving Size: 1 serving

Ingredients:

- 1/2 cup cottage cheese (low-fat)

- 1/2 cup cherry tomatoes, halved

- Salt and pepper, to taste

- Fresh basil leaves, for garnish (optional)

Instructions:

1. In a bowl, combine the cottage cheese and cherry tomatoes.

2. Season with salt and pepper to taste. Garnish with fresh basil leaves if desired.

3. Serve immediately as a refreshing and protein-packed snack.

Nutritional Information:

- Calories: 90
- Protein: 12g
- Carbohydrates: 6g
- Fat: 2g
- Fiber: 1g
- Sodium: 350mg

Advice for Social Events and Eating Out

Eating out and going to social gatherings may be challenging when trying to keep a balanced diet and make wise food choices. You may still enjoy these times and meet your nutritional goals, however, if you prepare ahead of time and make thoughtful decisions. Here are some guidelines for socializing and eating out:

Make a plan in advance:

- Examine the Menu in Advance: If at all possible, peruse the restaurant's menu online before your visit. Plan your meals and look for healthier options.

- Eat a Short Snack: To assist manage your hunger and avoid overindulging, enjoy a small, well-balanced snack before you leave.

Make Wise Choices:

- Select lean protein options that can be grilled, roasted, or steamed, such as fish, poultry, or tofu.

- To increase your intake of fiber, choose salads or vegetable-based meals as sides or main courses.

- Portion Control: Be mindful of the amounts you eat. Before you start eating, think about sharing an entrée with a friend or getting a to-go box so you can take half of your meal with you.

- Steer clear of fried or creamy options: Avoiding deep-fried and creamy dishes is advised due to their high calorie and saturated fat content.

- Select low-calorie beverages like water or herbal tea in place of sugary soft drinks.

Customize Your Purchase:

- Don't hesitate to adjust your order to suit your dietary requirements. Select grilled meals over fried ones, and order dressings and sauces on the side.

Watch What You Drink:

- Limit Your Alcohol Consumption: If alcohol is your preferred beverage, use it sparingly. Drinking alcohol may lower inhibitions and increase calorie intake, which can lead to poor eating decisions.
- To help control your appetite, stay hydrated throughout the meal by sipping water.

Use Smaller Plates and Practice Portion Control:

- Use a smaller dish during social occasions with buffets or finger snacks to help limit portion sizes.

Recognize When You're Hungry:

- Pay attention to your body's signals of hunger. Eat slowly, stopping when you're full but not full.

Social Services:

- Tell your friends and family what your nutritional goals are, and ask them to help you choose eateries and meals that fit your needs.

Intentional Eating:

- Appreciate Each Bite: When eating, take your time. You may find it easier to know when to stop eating if you eat slowly.

- Remain In the Moment: Attend to social interactions and dialogues rather than concentrating just on the food.

Snacks and Desserts:

- Desserts should be shared: If you're craving dessert, think about dividing it up with someone so you may each have a smaller portion.

- Make A Wise Choice: If fruit-based or reduced-calorie dessert options are available, consider them.

Moderate Exercise:

- While occasional indulgence is okay, moderation is crucial. You only need to consume your favorite meals and snacks less often and in smaller quantities rather than giving them up entirely.

Regarding Social Gatherings:

- Bring a Nutritious Dish: To ensure there is something nutrient-dense available at the potluck or party, bring a dish that you like that is healthy.

- Act Polite but Firm: Refuse meals or drinks that don't fit your dietary goals with grace. "No thank you, I'm trying to eat better," may be your response.

WORKOUT FOR ENDOMORPHS

The Benefits of Exercise for Endomorph Weight Management

Controlling weight is crucial for endomorphs. Compared to other body types, endomorphs may find it more difficult to lose weight or keep it off due to their innate tendency to gain fat. On the other hand, endomorphs may find that regular exercise is a very useful tool for managing their weight, maintaining general health, and reaching fitness goals. Exercise helps with endomorph weight control in the following ways:

Enhances the Metabolism:

Exercise may increase metabolism, particularly high-intensity interval training (HIIT) and strength training. Weight control is made easier by a quicker metabolic rate, which signifies that the body burns more calories during rest.

Burned Calories:

All forms of physical activity, including strength training regimens like weightlifting and cardiovascular exercises like running, burn calories. This burn of calories aids in weight loss or maintenance.

Boosts Muscular Mass:

Endomorphs need to engage in resistance training to gain and maintain lean muscle mass. Increasing muscle mass may help with long-term weight control since at rest, muscle burns more calories than fat does.

Promotes Fat Loss:

Frequent exercise improves the body's capacity to burn fat stores for energy, especially cardiovascular exercises. The proportion of total body fat may drop as a consequence.

Regulates Sensitivity to Insulin:

By increasing insulin sensitivity, exercise helps the body better regulate blood sugar levels. Better control of blood sugar may reduce the incidence of type 2 diabetes and prevent the accumulation of excess fat.

Results in Higher Energy Usage:

Engaging in physical activity increases daily energy expenditure, which helps achieve the necessary calorie deficit for weight reduction. This is particularly important for endomorphs since they tend to put on weight.

Enhanced Heart Health:

Regular aerobic exercise, like running, cycling, or swimming, may improve cardiovascular health and reduce the risk of heart disease, all of which are essential for overall well-being.

Helps Control Appetite:

Controlling hunger hormones with the help of exercise may help you better control food cravings and portion sizes.

Exercise improves motivation and mood:

Exercise releases endorphins, which may elevate motivation and mood. This is particularly helpful for endomorphs who could run into psychological problems while trying to lose weight.

Promotes Sustaining Weight Over Time:

Including exercise in your routine increases the likelihood that you will maintain your weight loss over the long run in addition to helping you lose weight.

Encourages a Healthier Way of Living:

Regular exercise is the cornerstone of a healthy lifestyle. It supports mental and physical health in addition to weight reduction.

For the best weight management, endomorphs should include a combination of strength, flexibility, and cardio exercises in their fitness regimen. Moreover, it is important to maintain consistency. In addition to exercise, a nutritious diet and overall lifestyle decisions are critical to effective weight control.

Developing an Exercise Program for Endomorphs

Exercise regimens for endomorphs should include strength training, flexibility training, and aerobic activity. Increasing lean muscle mass, fat loss, and metabolism are the goals. Here is a detailed process for designing a workout regimen tailored to endomorphs:

Determine Your Fitness Level: Before starting, determine your present level of fitness. This can help you determine the intensity of your exercises and help you create reasonable goals.

Establish Particular Goals: Specify clear, measurable, and doable goals. Setting clear goals for your exercise program may help you achieve weight loss, muscle growth, or improved cardiovascular health.

Integrate Strength and Cardiovascular Exercises: A comprehensive program should include both strength and cardiovascular exercises.

At least 150 minutes of moderate-intensity or 75 minutes of vigorous-intensity cardio should be done each week. You may go cycling, swimming, dancing, brisk walking, or running. Engaging in cardiovascular activity improves heart health and burns calories.

Incorporate strength training exercises into your routine at least twice a week. Complex exercises including squats, deadlifts, bench presses, and pull-ups train several muscle groups. Increased metabolism and fat loss are two benefits of lean muscle mass.

Circuit training and high-intensity interval training (HIIT): You should think about including any of these techniques in your exercise regimen. These exercises are efficient in improving fat loss and burning calories. They are made up of quick bursts of intense activity and quick rest periods in between.

Emphasize Core Strength: Endomorphs may be more likely to carry belly fat. Planks, Russian twists, and leg lifts are a few core-strengthening exercises that may help tone and tighten this region.

Incorporate Work Flexibility and Mobility: To improve flexibility and prevent injuries, regular mobility exercises and stretches should be performed. Endomorphs benefit greatly from yoga and pilates classes since they improve body awareness and flexibility.

Prioritize Consistency: Maintaining and achieving fitness goals requires consistency. Make exercise a regular part of your routine and choose activities you like to help you remain motivated.

Track Progress: Use fitness tracking apps or maintain a workout journal to gauge your progress. Maintaining a record of your workouts, weight, body measurements, and other relevant information can assist you in staying on course and making any necessary program adjustments.

Nutrition and hydration: Exercise is not enough to maintain a healthy weight on its own. Eat a balanced diet and drink plenty of water. It's crucial to maintain a nutritious diet that complements your fitness goals.

Rest and Recovery: Allow your body to rest and recover after each session. Resting enough is essential for overall health and muscle repair.

Have Patience: Remember that progress takes time. Try your hardest, be patient, and don't allow little setbacks to demotivate you.

Cardiovascular Endomorph Workouts

Exercises that target the heart are a crucial component of an endomorph fitness regimen. You may reduce weight, improve your cardiovascular health, and burn calories with these activities. The following effective cardiovascular exercises are tailored especially for endomorphs:

Walking quickly: Most people may get low-impact cardiovascular exercise by brisk walking. It's a fantastic choice for beginners and those who want to gradually introduce a workout schedule.

Try to get in at least 30 minutes of brisk walking most days of the week. Increase the duration and intensity progressively as your fitness level rises.

Running or jogging: These activities are more strenuous forms of cardiovascular training. It may help you increase your cardiovascular fitness and lose weight.

If you've never run before, begin with the run-walk technique. As your endurance increases, try going on longer, continuous runs.

Include interval training by alternating between faster running periods and slower recovery jogging intervals to enhance calorie burn.

Riding a bike: Riding a bike, either outdoors or on a stationary cycle, is a good way to strengthen your legs and increase your heart rate.

One way to employ interval training is to ride hard for short bursts of time, and then recover at a lower effort level.

Swimming: Working the whole body, swimming is a low-impact cardiovascular exercise. It's ideal for endomorphs who are worried about joint impact since it's gentle on the joints.

Increase the amount of calories burned by swimming laps at a moderate to fast pace.

Dancing: Dancing-based workouts, like Zumba or dance aerobics, are an enjoyable and effective way to increase your heart rate.

You may express yourself via dancing and improve your cardiovascular endurance with these exercises.

Elliptical Machine: An elliptical machine may provide a full-body, low-impact workout that is easy on the joints.

By changing the resistance and slope, you may intensify your exercise.

Climbing the Stairs: Whether you're using a stair climber machine or regular stairs, climbing steps is a fantastic way to strengthen your legs and increase your heart rate.

It's a vigorous exercise that may increase cardiovascular fitness and help you burn calories.

High-intensity interval training, or HIIT, comprises brief sessions of high-intensity exercise interspersed with brief rest periods. This approach has the potential to improve cardiovascular fitness and aid with weight loss.

Cardiovascular activities such as running, cycling, and bodyweight exercises like burpees and jumping jacks may all be done with HIIT.

Group Exercise Classes: Taking part in group exercise classes, like aerobics, kickboxing, or spinning, may help you mix up your cardio routine and foster social interactions.

Engage in outdoor recreation by taking part in sports like basketball or tennis, or by hiking or trail running. These workouts might benefit your heart in addition to being enjoyable.

Tone Your Muscles with Strength Training

Any fitness program that tries to acquire a more toned physique and build muscle tone must include strength training. Strength training may help you acquire muscle tone by growing muscle mass and lowering body fat. Muscle tone is defined as the

firmness and definition of your muscles. Here's how to create a
strength training program for muscular tone:

Identify Your Goals:

- Specify your exact goals for muscular tone. Do you want to target certain muscle groups, like your arms, legs, or core, or your whole body? Setting clear objectives will help you design a successful exercise program.

Choose the Right Exercises:

- Mix up your routines with both isolation and complex exercises. Exercises that work many muscle groups simultaneously, such as squats, deadlifts, and bench presses, are excellent for building overall muscular tone. Exercises that isolate certain muscles, like leg extensions and bicep curls, may help define those muscles.

Establish a Split Routine:

- Split your strength training sessions across several body areas or muscle groups to get balanced growth and recovery. A common split program involves working on various muscular groups on different days, such as the arms, legs, chest, and back.

Repetition and Resistance:

- Choose the appropriate level of resistance for every activity. You should feel challenged yet still be able to complete your repetitions with the correct technique.
- For every exercise, 2-4 sets of 8–15 repetitions are optimal. Increasing the number of repetitions while using lighter weights may help build muscle tone and endurance.

Gradual Overload:

- Increase the resistance (weights) or repetitions gradually as your strength and endurance improve. This progressive strain is essential for the growth and tone of muscles.

Full Range of Motion:

- Perform each exercise through its full range of motion to fully activate the target muscles. Steer clear of momentum and swinging while lifting weights.

Rest and recovery:

- Give yourself ample time in between muscle groups and sets. Muscles need time to develop and recover.
- Give yourself at least 48 hours in between workouts targeting the same muscle area.

Incorporate Core Exercises:

- Stability and proper muscle tone depend on a strong core. Incorporate exercises that engage your core muscles, such as leg lifts, Russian twists, and planks.

Combine strength and cardio training:

- Combining strength and cardio training will assist lower body fat percentage overall and highlight the toned muscles below.

Appropriate Nutrition:

- To support muscle growth and repair, give your body a well-balanced diet high in protein. Ensure that you consume enough calories to maintain your current level of activity and your desired amount of muscle growth.

Consistency:

- Increasing muscle tone requires consistency. Continue your strength training program and challenge your muscles progressively.

Form and Technique:

- Use proper form and technique for every exercise to minimize the risk of injury and to get the best possible results. Seeking to ensure ideal form or being new to strength training, you may wish to work with a professional personal trainer.

Flexibility and Mobility:

- To improve flexibility and lower your risk of injury, include mobility exercises and stretches in your routine.

WORKOUT PLANS

This exercise program is designed to complement the meal plan, focusing on burning fat, building muscle, and improving overall fitness for beginners, specially tailored for endomorph body types. The program includes a mix of cardiovascular training, strength training, and flexibility exercises to provide a well-rounded approach.

Week 1 & 2: Foundation Building

Day 1: Full Body Strength Training

- Warm-up: 5-minute brisk walk or jog

- Circuit (Repeat 2x):

    - Squats: 12 reps

    - Push-ups (knees, if necessary): 10 reps

    - Dumbbell Rows: 12 reps each side

    - Plank: 30 seconds

- Cool down: Stretching, 5 minutes

Day 2: Cardio + Core

- Warm-up: 5-minute brisk walk

- Cardio: 20-minute walk or jog

- Core Circuit (Repeat 2x):

    - Russian Twists: 15 reps on each side

    - Bicycle Crunches: 15 reps on each side

    - Leg Raises: 10 reps

- Cool down: Stretching, 5 minutes

Day 3: Active Recovery

- Activities: 30-minute walk, yoga, or light swimming

Day 4: Lower Body Strength

- Warm-up: 5-minute brisk walk or jog

- Circuit (Repeat 2x):

    - Lunges: 10 reps for each leg

    - Deadlifts (use dumbbells): 12 reps

    - Calf Raises: 15 reps

    - Glute Bridges: 12 reps

- Cool down: Stretching, 5 minutes

Day 5: Cardio Interval Training

- Warm-up: 5-minute walk

- Interval Training: Alternate 1-minute jog with 2 minutes walk for 20 minutes

- Cool down: Stretching, 5 minutes

Day 6: Upper Body Strength

- Warm-up: 5-minute brisk walk or jog

- Circuit (Repeat 2x):

    - Shoulder Press: 12 reps

    - Tricep Dips: 10 reps

    - Bicep Curls: 12 reps for each arm

    - Side Planks: 20 seconds on each side

- Cool down: Stretching, 5 minutes

Day 7: Rest or Light Activity

- Activities: Gentle walk, stretching, or rest

Week 3 & 4: Intensity Increase

Day 1: Full Body Strength Training

- Increase circuit to 3x with moderate weights

Day 2: Cardio + Core

- Increase Cardio to 30 minutes

- Add set to the Core Circuit

Day 3: Active Recovery

- Include dynamic stretching or a beginner's yoga session

Day 4: Lower Body Strength

- Increase circuit to 3x; consider adding weight for more challenge

Day 5: HIIT Cardio

- 25 minutes of HIIT: 30 seconds sprint, 1 minute walk

Day 6: Upper Body Strength

- Increase circuit to 3x; adjust weights to maintain challenge

Day 7: Rest or Active Recovery

- Choose a recovery activity that you enjoy

Key Points:

- **Warm up** before and **cool down** after every workout.

- **Stay hydrated** and listen to your body, adjusting intensity as needed.

- **Rest days** are crucial for recovery; don't skip them.

- **Progressive overload:** As you grow stronger, gradually increase the weights or reps to continue challenging your body.

- **Flexibility work** such as stretching or yoga is vital for recovery and injury prevention; incorporate it regularly.

The Relationship Between Evolution and Adaptation

Progression and adaptation are key concepts in the study of fitness and exercise science. Whether your goals are to gain more strength and endurance, lose weight, or enhance your overall health, these concepts are critical to achieving and maintaining your fitness goals. In the context of exercise, progression and adaptation function as follows:

Progression:

- Gradual Overload: The technique of gradually increasing the demands placed on your body during physical activity is known as progression. This is known as "progressive overload" at times. By pushing your body beyond its current limits, you encourage it to adapt and grow stronger or more efficient.

- Increasing Intensity: By making your exercises more intense, you may advance. This might include increasing the resistance on cardio equipment, running further or faster, or lifting heavier weights.

- More Reps or Sets: Adding more sets or repetitions to your strength training exercises is another way to become bigger. For instance, you may go up to three sets of 12 repetitions or more if you've been doing three sets of 10 reps for a certain exercise.

- Frequency: Increasing the number of times you work out might aid in your personal development. This means adding additional sessions or working out more often each week.

- Modify: Adapting training plans, exercise routines, or training modalities might be seen as progress. Try cycling for a bit if you've been running, for instance, to build new muscle groups and prevent plateaus.

Adaptation:

- Physiological Changes: Your body adapts to increasing demands by going through physiological changes as it is continuously exposed to increasing overload. Among the benefits are enhanced neuromuscular coordination, greater cardiovascular efficiency, enhanced muscle strength, and increased endurance.

- Better Performance: Performance improves as a result of adaptation. Exercises that you found challenging before will become easier, enabling you to run faster, lift heavier weights, and complete more repetitions with less effort.

- Preventing Plateaus: Consistent progress and adaptation are necessary to prevent plateaus in your fitness path. When your body stops improving and becomes used to a certain level of stress, a plateau occurs. By increasing the intensity or varying your routines, you may avoid these training plateaus.

- Injury Prevention: Appropriate development and adaptability also help to avoid injuries. Your body has time to strengthen the muscles, ligaments, and joints as it gradually adjusts to new demands, which reduces the likelihood of overuse issues.

- Long-Term Success: Adaptability and growth are essential for long-term fitness success. Whether your objectives are short- or long-term, following these principles can help you remain on course and get the benefits of consistent exercise.

- Periodization is a great way to include flexibility and advancement. This is a methodical training approach where you divide your training into many stages, each with a distinct focus on volume, intensity, and choice of activities. Periodization contributes to result optimization, minimizes the risk of burnout, and prevents overtraining.

Cross-training and variation

A well-rounded approach to achieving your fitness and health goals involves cross-training and adding variety to your training routine. By using these techniques, you may reduce your chance of overuse injuries, stay off plateaus, and maintain a fun and engaging training regimen. The following are some ways that diversification and cross-training might benefit your fitness journey:

Cross-Training:

Cross-training means doing a variety of different types of physical activity or exercise instead of focusing mostly on one. You may concentrate on different muscle groups, energy systems, and movement patterns with its help. The following are a few benefits of cross-training:

- Overuse Injuries: Daily repetition of the same workouts or movements might result in overuse injuries. By exercising certain muscle regions while resting others, cross-training reduces the chance of overuse problems.
- Muscle Development: Varied exercises put different demands on various muscle groups. By encouraging

healthy muscle development, cross-training reduces the risk of muscular imbalances, which may result in injuries or poor posture.

- Increasing Total Fitness: You may increase your total fitness by engaging in a range of activities that will improve your physical strength, flexibility, agility, and cardiovascular endurance.

- Cross-training helps to maintain your motivation and intellectual engagement by providing a mental respite from the monotony of the same program.

- Adaptation and Progression: Your body must adapt to new challenges as you switch up your activities. You may improve your performance in your primary sport or workout regimen with this adaption.

Variety:

Diversity within a certain fitness regimen, like strength training or aerobic classes, may also be beneficial. The following are some ways that adding diversity to your fitness regimen might help:

- Muscle Confusion: By periodically modifying your training regimen or exercises, you may prevent your muscles from adapting too quickly.

- By sticking to the same routines or exercises, boredom may be avoided and muscle growth and strength can be enhanced. Training sessions become more engaging and enjoyable when they are varied.

- Diverse exercises are more beneficial for reaching different fitness goals. For instance, one may use isolated exercises to define muscles and intricate routines to increase strength.

- Discovering Hobbies: Having a variety of experiences encourages you to try new things and discover interests outside of fitness. You could find that you like pastimes you've never thought of before.

Cross-training and many illustrations:

In addition to running, cardiovascular exercise may include activities like cycling, swimming, hiking, or rowing.

Change up your strength training routine by using different equipment, rep ranges, and exercises. Included should be machine exercises, resistance bands, free weights, and bodyweight exercises.

Yoga, Pilates, and static stretching may be used to increase flexibility and mobility.

High-Intensity Interval Training (HIIT): Varied HIIT regimens with distinct intervals and exercises are performed.

Take part in your favorite sports or pastimes, such as martial arts, basketball, tennis, or dancing.

Participate in a variety of group fitness classes, including dance aerobics, kickboxing, spinning, and barre.

SLEEP AND RECOVERY

Relaxation is Crucial for Endomorphs

For endomorphs as for persons of all body types, rest is essential. Enough rest and recovery are essential components of an effective and well-balanced exercise and weight-control plan. For endomorphs, relaxing is crucial for the following reasons:

Regeneration of Muscle:

For endomorphs as well as other fitness regimes, strength training is a crucial part. Your muscle fibers sustain microtears when you lift weights or work out with resistance. Rest periods provide these tears the time they need to repair and replenish. Your muscles won't be able to repair and grow if you don't get enough sleep, which might result in overtraining and injury.

Balance of Hormones:

Hormone balance is maintained via rest, and this is crucial for both general health and weight control. Your body produces growth hormone when you sleep, and this hormone is crucial for fat metabolism, muscle development, and overall healing. Rest or sleep deprivation may throw off your hormone balance and make it harder for you to lose weight.

Preventing Overuse Injuries:

Endomorphs are susceptible to overuse injuries just like everyone else if they don't allow their bodies enough time to heal. When muscles and joints are repeatedly strained without enough recovery, overuse problems may result. Different training regimens and rest days help to avoid certain illnesses.

Recovering Energy:

Exercise regularly may be physically taxing, particularly for endomorphs attempting to reduce weight. Rest days enable your body to replenish energy reserves like glycogen, giving you the endurance to complete your exercises.

Restoration of the Mind:

Not only is sleep essential for physical recovery, but it also promotes mental wellness. A well-rounded workout plan allows for recovery and mental rejuvenation periods. An excessive amount of training may lead to stress, low motivation, and mental tiredness. Rest allows your mind to clear and keeps you inspired to continue on your fitness journey.

Immune System Assistance:

A lengthy period of intense exercise may momentarily weaken the immune system. Getting enough sleep helps your body heal and strengthens your immune system, which reduces the likelihood of illness and makes it easier for you to maintain a regular workout regimen.

Extended-Term Growth:

Getting enough sleep is essential for long-term success. Regular rest days and recuperation periods make maintaining consistency in your fitness program easier. This lessens tiredness and increases the likelihood that you will eventually reach your fitness and weight reduction goals.

Tips for Rest and Recuperation

- Rest Days: Assemble a weekly training schedule that includes regular rest days. You may either do nothing but relax or take part in low-impact exercises like yoga or walking on these days.

- Get 7 to 9 hours of good sleep each night to support overall health and muscle recovery.

- To increase blood flow and aid in recovery, consider doing easy, low-impact workouts like foam rolling, stretching, or gentle cycling on your days off.

- Pay attention to what you eat, particularly what you eat after an exercise. A healthy diet provides your muscles with the essential nutrients they need to repair.

- Pay Attention to Your Body: Prolonged fatigue, subpar performance, and heightened vulnerability to illness are signs of overtraining. If necessary, increase the intensity of your exercises or schedule more days off.

- Drink plenty of water throughout the day since dehydration may impair performance and recuperation.

Techniques for Successful Recuperation

Individuals who exercise regularly, athletes, and people of all activity levels need to know how to properly recover from injuries. A healthy recovery process enhances performance, prevents overuse injuries, and advances overall well-being. Here are a few successful recuperation techniques:

Rest and sleep: Aim for seven to nine hours of good sleep each night and make sleep a priority. Our bodies repair and regenerate tissues, control hormones, and strengthen memory and learning when we sleep.

Intense Rehabilitation: Incorporate light, low-impact activity on rest days. Exercises like swimming, light yoga, and walking may aid with recovery by easing muscle tension, increasing blood flow, and promoting relaxation.

Flexibility and stretching: To improve flexibility and reduce muscle tension, do static stretches after an exercise. Focus on your main muscle groups and hold each stretch for 15-30 seconds.

Self-Massage and Foam Rolling: Use a massage stick or foam roller to work on tense or sore muscles. This self-myofascial release technique helps improve blood flow and relax tense muscles.

Hydration: Drink plenty of water throughout the day. Hydration is essential for proper muscular contraction, the transfer of nutrients, and overall healing.

Nutrition: To support muscle growth and repair, eat a well-balanced diet high in protein. To replenish glycogen stores and aid in recovery, have a post-workout breakfast or snack that includes both carbohydrates and protein.

Heat and Ice Therapy: Apply ice to sore or inflammatory areas to reduce swelling and discomfort (cryotherapy). Applying a warm compress or other kind of heat treatment, or thermotherapy, may help relax muscles and improve blood flow.

Compression Wear: Wearing compression sleeves or clothes helps enhance blood flow, lessen soreness in the muscles, and perhaps hasten the healing process.

Nutritional Timing: Eat a balanced breakfast or snack that includes both carbohydrates and protein between 30 minutes and two hours after working out to improve muscle repair.

Contrasting baths or showers: You may improve blood flow and reduce muscle soreness by dipping limbs in hot and cold water or switching between hot and cold water in the shower.

Professional healing modalities: If you're looking for more concentrated pain relief and healing, you may want to look into chiropractic, acupuncture, or massage therapy as professional recovery techniques.

Mental Relaxation: Practice relaxation methods like deep breathing exercises, mindfulness, or meditation to lower stress and promote mental healing.

Prevent Overtraining: Pay attention to your body and steer clear of too demanding training regimens since they might result in overtraining. Work rest days into your training schedule.

Periodization: Cycle through periods of different volumes and intensities throughout your training to improve recovery and adaptability.

Gradual Overload: To give your body time to adjust and recover in between sessions, gradually increase the volume and intensity of your workouts.

Track Your Progress: Maintain a training journal to record your workouts, nutritional intake, and recovery techniques. Adapt your plan as needed depending on how you're doing and how your body responds.

Stress Reduction and Sleep Quality

General health and well-being are largely dependent on getting enough sleep and managing stress. Both have a significant impact on one's quality of life, productivity, fitness, and mental and physical health, among other aspects of life. Here's how to effectively manage stress, sleep, and priorities:

Regulating Sleep:

- **Make Sleep a Priority:** Include sleep as much as possible in your daily routine. Aim for 7-9 hours of quality sleep each night to give your body the time it needs to unwind, heal, and repair.

- **Keep a Regular Sleep Schedule:** Go to bed and get up at the same hour every day, including on the weekends. Your body's internal clock may be regulated with the help of consistency.

- **Create a Sleep-Friendly Environment:** Keep your bedroom calm, cold, and dark to promote healthy sleep. If needed, think about using white noise generators and blackout drapes.

- **Cut Down on Screen Time:** Give yourself at least an hour before bed to avoid using screens, including phones, tablets, computers, and TVs. Blue light from screens may disrupt your body's production of the hormone melatonin, which controls sleep.

- **Relaxation Techniques:** Read a book, do mild yoga, or engage in meditation before retiring to bed. These breathing techniques may help you clear your mind and get your body ready for sleep.

- **Keep a Healthy Diet:** Avoid large meals, coffee, and alcohol just before bed. These may disrupt your sleeping patterns.

- **Engage in regular exercise:** Exercise regularly may improve your quality of sleep. On the other hand, avoiding strenuous activities too close to sleep may have the opposite effect.

- **Limitation on Naps:** To avoid interfering with your nocturnal sleep, limit your naps to 20 to 30 minutes and take them early in the day.

- **Stress Management:** Sleep disturbances may result from stress. Apply stress-reduction strategies to address this problem.

Reducing Stress:

- **Identify Stressors:** Take stock of the things that are causing you stress. Challenges in work, relationships, finances, and health are a few instances of this.

- **Time Management:** Prioritize your tasks, set reasonable goals, and use your time well. Having good time management reduces the emotions of overload.

- **Mindfulness and meditation:** These techniques may help you remain in the present moment and reduce worry. These methods might help you manage your stress right now.

- **Physical Activity:** Engaging in regular exercise releases endorphins, which are the body's natural mood boosters, and help reduce stress.

- **Social Relationships:** Keep your friends and family near to your heart. Seeking support and having a conversation with loved ones may be quite beneficial during trying times.

- **Relaxation Techniques:** Try deep breathing exercises, gradual muscle relaxation, or guided visualization to calm your mind and reduce tension.

- **Set Boundaries:** To protect your own time and space, set boundaries. Understand when to say no.

- **A Healthy Way of Life:** Prioritize self-care activities like hobbies and leisure, maintain a balanced diet, and engage in regular exercise to maintain overall well-being.

- **Sleep:** As mentioned earlier, it is important to prioritize good sleep hygiene since inadequate sleep may exacerbate stress.

Sleep and stress management must be balanced to maintain both physical and mental well-being. You can live a better life, perform better, and maintain psychological stability with the aid of these approaches. Try out several strategies to see what suits you the best, and remember that it's always a good idea to get professional assistance if you're having trouble sleeping or managing stress.

ALTERNATIVE ADVANCEMENT

Endomorph Supplements

Like persons of any body type, endomorphs may gain from taking supplements when combined with a balanced diet and regular exercise. They ought to help you achieve your entire fitness and health goals. Endomorphs may find the following dietary supplements beneficial:

Protein supplements: To help them meet their needs for protein, which is essential for muscle growth and repair, endomorphs may benefit from taking protein supplements such as whey, casein, or plant-based protein. Smoothies with protein might be a simple post-workout snack.

Branched-Chain Amino Acids (BCAAs): Leucine, isoleucine, and valine make up BCAAs, which may aid in muscle regeneration and pain management. People who engage in demanding exercises and strength training often use them.

Fat Compounds Omega-3: Supplements containing omega-3 fatty acids, such as fish oil or algae oil (for vegans and vegetarians), may lower inflammation, strengthen the heart, and perhaps even assist with weight loss.

Vitamin D Deficiency: Endomorphs may be among the many individuals who lack this nutrient. Immune system performance, bone health, and overall well-being all depend on vitamin D. Think about getting your vitamin D levels evaluated and taking supplements if necessary.

Calcium: Endomorphs, who are more inclined to carry excess weight that puts stress on the bones, may benefit particularly from calcium, which is crucial for bone health.

Magnesium (Mg): Maintaining bone health, energy production, and muscle and neuron function are all aided by magnesium. It could help relax muscles and reduce cramping.

Supplemental Fiber: Although fiber is best absorbed via complete meals, endomorphs who have trouble controlling their weight or with digestion can find that a supplement helps.

Green Tea Extract: This extract contains compounds including catechins and antioxidants that may help with metabolism and weight loss. Although it is not a miraculous treatment, it may be used in conjunction with other weight-loss techniques.

Pre-Workout Supplements: Common ingredients in pre-workout supplements include caffeine, beta-alanine, and precursors to nitric oxide. They may enhance athletic performance and provide an energy boost. However because some individuals are sensitive to stimulants, they should be used with care.

Multivitamins: Making sure you get the vitamins and minerals required for overall health by taking a high-quality multivitamin will help fill in any nutritional gaps in your diet.

Probiotics: Good gut health is essential for proper digestion, metabolism, and overall well-being. Maintaining a healthy gut might aid with weight reduction.

Hormones and Controlling Weight

Hormones have a major role in both general health and weight control. Making informed choices regarding your diet, exercise routine, and way of life is made possible by having a better understanding of how hormones affect your body. The following key hormones have an impact on controlling weight:

The pancreatic hormone insulin regulates blood sugar levels. It facilitates the removal of glucose from the bloodstream for either fat storage or energy use. Weight gain is a common side effect of insulin resistance, which is the ineffective response of cells to insulin and is associated with conditions like type 2 diabetes.

The "satiety hormone" is leptin, which signals to your brain that you've eaten enough and should quit eating. In some situations, the brain may not react to leptin signals, which may result in leptin resistance and perhaps contribute to overeating and weight gain.

Ghrelin: The stomach produces ghrelin, sometimes known as the "hunger hormone." It stimulates hunger and signals to the brain when it's time to eat. Overindulgence in food and weight gain may result from elevated ghrelin levels.

Cortisol: In response to stress, the body produces cortisol, sometimes referred to as the "stress hormone." Prolonged stress may increase cortisol levels, which can lead to weight gain, particularly visceral fat.

Thyroid hormones: Thyroid hormones, namely T3 and T4, are crucial for controlling metabolism. When the thyroid gland does not produce enough thyroid hormones, the disease known as hypothyroidism may lead to weight gain and difficulty losing weight.

The sex hormones progesterone and estrogen might affect how well a person manages their weight. Hormonal illnesses, menopause, and changes in hormone levels throughout the menstrual cycle may all affect a woman's ability to regulate her weight.

Testosterone: Although it is present in smaller levels in females, testosterone is the primary sex hormone in men. Low testosterone levels may cause weight gain, a slower metabolism, and muscle loss in both men and women.

Growth hormone (GH): Growth hormone stimulates the metabolism of fat and the development of muscles. Low GH levels, which are often associated with aging, may cause weight gain and muscle atrophy.

The hormone adiponectin is produced by fat cells and helps control insulin sensitivity and metabolism. Low levels of adiponectin are associated with obesity and insulin resistance.

Catecholamines: Norepinephrine and adrenaline: These hormones are produced during the "fight or flight" stress response and can momentarily increase energy expenditure and metabolism.

How to Control Your Hormones to Lose Weight:

- Balanced Diet: Consume a diet rich in a variety of nutrients and well-balanced to help with hormone regulation. Meals high in fiber, lean proteins, and healthy fats may all support stable blood sugar levels.

- Engage in regular exercise to improve metabolism, lower stress levels, and insulin sensitivity.

- Stress Reduction: To manage cortisol levels, engage in stress-reduction techniques including mindfulness, deep breathing, and meditation.

- Sufficient Sleep: Prioritize getting enough sleep since insufficient sleep may throw off hormone balance and make you feel more hungry.

- Hormone Replacement Therapy: In some cases, treating hormonal abnormalities may need hormone replacement therapy administered under a doctor's supervision.

- Frequent Health Checkups: Routine health examinations may assist in identifying and treating hormone imbalances or other medical conditions.

IN CONCLUSION

All things considered, "The Extreme Endomorph Diet and Exercise Plan for Beginners" is a thorough manual designed especially for those with endomorphic body types. We've examined the unique obstacles that endomorphs encounter on their fitness journeys in this book and offered helpful advice to assist them get beyond these obstacles and meet their wellness and health goals.

We started our adventure with a thorough explanation of endomorph body types, emphasizing the value of recognizing individual variances and the impact of heredity on our physical characteristics. Knowing their specific body type gives endomorphs the ability to make well-informed choices about their food and exercise regimen.

The value of customized techniques has been a recurrent subject in the book. We've made it clear that there isn't a one-size-fits-all approach to exercise and wellness. Rather, endomorphs have to modify their strategies to suit their unique requirements, inclinations, and objectives.

We've covered the traits that distinguish endomorphs, such as their rounder build, slower metabolism, and tendency to accumulate fat. This knowledge is a fundamental component in creating diet and activity plans that work.

We've looked at the process of creating health and fitness targets to set the stage for a successful fitness journey. The need to establish specific, attainable, quantifiable goals that take into account both short- and long-term objectives has been emphasized.

One key has been establishing reasonable objectives that are appropriate for the endomorph body type. We've covered how to set realistic goals for building muscle, losing weight, and improving your general health. Setting and maintaining objectives that inspire and last throughout time has been emphasized.

Keeping track of our progress and staying motivated have been crucial components of our trip. We've spoken about several ways to monitor your fitness progress, such as journaling or using modern fitness devices. Various approaches have been proposed to address the issue of staying motivated, including seeking responsibility, acknowledging accomplishments, and embracing a growth-oriented attitude.

The book's main focus is its thorough analysis of endomorph nutrition and food planning. We have discussed the dietary needs that are unique to endomorphs, including macronutrient ratios, calorie control, and the need for meals high in nutrients. The book provides thorough guidance on creating an endomorph diet plan that addresses topics including portion management, meal planning, and encouraging long-lasting good eating habits.

To help endomorphs make healthy choices, we've included example weekly meal plans that demonstrate how these dietary guidelines might be put into practice.

We've put up a selection of breakfast, lunch, and dinner meals with detailed directions and nutritional data for individuals looking for a wide variety of recipes. These dishes are not only delicious, but they are also thoughtfully designed to assist endomorphs in reaching their fitness and weight loss goals.

Practical advice on handling social gatherings and eating out has been provided to enable endomorphs to make health-conscious choices while enjoying social interactions.

Now that we've covered the exercise part, let's talk about how important it is for endomorph weight control. We've assisted endomorphs in creating a customized fitness program that includes aerobic, strength, and flexibility training.

We've covered more ground in the core ideas of progression, adaptability, cross-training, and variation to make sure endomorphs keep their bodies challenged all the time, avoiding plateaus and overuse issues.

We have now discussed the importance of rest and recovery as well as practical recovery techniques. We have emphasized the need to get enough sleep for hormone balance, muscle repair, and general health. There have been detailed rehabilitation plans that involve self-care routines, stress reduction, and sleep management.

"The Extreme Endomorph Diet and Exercise Plan for Beginners" is essentially a comprehensive guide that provides endomorphs with the information, resources, and tactics needed to make a successful transition to improved health and fitness. Endomorphs may achieve their fitness objectives and live a better and more energetic life by adopting customized strategies, establishing realistic goals, making educated food choices, and exercising regularly. Recall that the secret to success is not just getting where you're going, but also enjoying the trip, where every step you take is a step closer to better health and wellbeing.

www.ingramcontent.com/pod-product-compliance
Lightning Source LLC
Chambersburg PA
CBHW050816260726
48660CB00004B/1465